From Patient to Advocate

Turning Survivorship Into Impact
A Healthcare Advocate's Guide

Tim McDonald

ISBN: 979-8-9947103-0-2

First Edition, 2026

Printed in the United States of America

To my wife, Lori, who has stood by my side through every step of this journey, supporting my advocacy work with unwavering love and understanding. Your belief in me made all of this possible.

To my fellow advocates, those still fighting alongside me and those who have passed but whose wisdom and courage I carry with me every day. You inspire me to keep going.

To my friends who made this journey not just bearable, but meaningful. Without you, I don't know how we would have done it.

And to Man Up To Cancer, Fight CRC, and COLONTOWN, the organizations that didn't just start my advocacy journey, but wrapped their arms around me after my diagnosis and showed me what community truly means.

Acknowledgments

This book exists because of the countless advocates, patients, caregivers, and healthcare professionals who have generously shared their time, wisdom, and experiences with me over the past five years.

To the advocacy organizations that have given me opportunities to learn, grow, and serve. Fight Colorectal Cancer, Man Up To Cancer, COLONTOWN, Hematology/Oncology Pharmacy Association (HOPA), PAN Foundation, and Patient-Centered Outcomes Research Institute (PCORI), thank you for trusting me with leadership roles and for the incredible support you've provided not just to me, but to countless others navigating their advocacy journeys.

To the listeners of the Advocacy at Work podcast and readers of my Substack, your engagement and questions helped shape this book into something truly useful for the advocacy community.

To every advocate I've met at conferences, retreats, and online communities, your stories and strategies fill these pages. This guide is as much yours as it is mine.

And finally, to Lori, whose patience during countless hours of writing, editing, and advocacy work never wavered. Your support made this book, and this life, possible.

Abbreviations

The following abbreviations are used throughout this book:

Fight CRC: Fight Colorectal Cancer

HOPA: Hematology/Oncology Pharmacy Association

PAN Foundation: Patient Access Network Foundation

PCORI: Patient-Centered Outcomes Research Institute

COLONTOWN: Online support community for colorectal cancer patients

CDMRP: Congressionally Directed Medical Research Programs

RATS: Research Advocacy Training and Support (Fight CRC program)

CRC: Colorectal Cancer

Contents

Chapter 1

What is Advocacy?
Defining Your Why

The Day Everything Changed

I'll never forget the moment the doctor said, "You have cancer." I was 52 years old. It was November 2020, and the world was locked down. I had no family history of colorectal cancer. I did all the things you're supposed to do. I ate well. I exercised. I attended regular checkups. And then one day, I had pain in my right flank. What started as a quick urgent care visit turned into a CT scan, a colonoscopy, and a diagnosis that would change everything.

Stage IV colorectal cancer. The kind that had already spread to my liver.

What I didn't know in that moment was that this diagnosis would eventually lead to a calling far greater than myself. I didn't know that within a few years, I'd be sitting on research steering committees, reviewing grant proposals for the Department of Defense, mentoring newly diagnosed patients, testifying before state legislators, and speaking at conferences about patient advocacy. I didn't know that I'd receive a liver transplant from a living donor and dedicate myself to helping other metastatic colorectal cancer patients find donors through ShareMyLiver.com. I also didn't know the full spectrum of what was possible.

When you're newly diagnosed with cancer, or other chronic disease, people tell you a lot of things. Family members tell you to stay positive. Friends tell you to fight. Other patients tell you about support groups and therapists. Some of them suggest getting involved with patient organizations. Maybe volunteer, they say. It'll help you process everything. That's what I did when I applied to become an ambassador with Fight CRC, an organization dedicated to colorectal cancer prevention, research, and support.

But once I got there, I was exposed to something I didn't expect. There were all these different ways to get involved. Awareness work. Research advocacy. Legislative advocacy. Fundraising. These weren't just volunteer positions. They were different paths to creating actual change.

Naturally, I gravitated toward what was familiar. I'd spent my entire career as a community manager, building connections and telling stories. Awareness work felt like home. But something interesting happened over time. I started exploring the other areas. I discovered I didn't need a research or science background to get involved with research advocacy. I just needed to listen carefully to what patients actually needed and communicate that perspective to researchers designing studies. I learned that working with legislators on issues affecting colorectal cancer patients filled my soul in ways I didn't expect. And I realized pretty quickly that, even though I'd been good at grassroots fundraising earlier in my career, I was already asking too much of my friends and professional network.

These discoveries pushed me beyond just raising awareness into some-thing far more strategic and impactful. They led me to healthcare advocacy.

What Advocacy Actually Is

Advocacy is one of those words that gets thrown around so much it sometimes loses meaning. People talk about "advocating" for almost anything. But in healthcare, when we talk about patient advocacy, we're talking about something much more specific and powerful.

Let me start with what it's not. Advocacy is not just volunteering.

Volunteering is important. Volunteering keeps nonprofits running. Volunteering connects people to community. But volunteering often operates within existing systems and structures. A volunteer might staff a helpline, organize an event, or coordinate communications. These are valuable roles, but they're not necessarily advocacy.

Advocacy is different. Advocacy is about influence, voice, and change. The Journal of Cancer Policy defines advocacy as the act of representing and pleading on behalf of patients to ensure their rights are upheld and improve access to quality treatment and care.1 These discoveries pushed me beyond just raising awareness into something far more strategic and impactful. They led me to healthcare advocacy. Working to change systems, influence policy, and shape research.

But it means something different to different people. And I think that's actually one of its greatest strengths.

I've had the privilege of working alongside advocates who each have their own way of articulating what advocacy means. Jon Brent, a fellow cancer advocate, describes it as being the bridge between silence and action, turning pain into power. There's something profound in that. It acknowledges both the starting point—silence, pain —and the destination: action and empowerment.

Dale Brooks frames it as sharing real, teachable, and actionable information. For Dale, advocacy is fundamentally about communication.

It's about making sure patients and communities have what they need to make informed decisions about their own care and lives.

Rodney Warner brings a different lens. His definition is about ensuring someone's wants, interests, and rights are met, especially when they're unable to communicate those things themselves. This speaks to the protective, sometimes fierce element of advocacy that shows up in every form—whether you're advocating for policy change, better research design, or individual patient needs. It's about standing up for those who can't stand up for themselves.

Rob Gurganious offers a more holistic view. He sees advocacy as helping patients get the most out of themselves, their medical teams, insurance, and any resources they have available. He does this by listening closely, lightening their load when possible, and fostering a sense of camaraderie and understanding in their struggles.

Dan Edwards keeps it simple and powerful. He defines advocacy as standing for yourself or someone else when no one else will. There's a clarity in that. Sometimes advocacy is just about not staying silent.

And for me, after years of working in this field, I believe that advocacy is as simple as sharing your story. Your story becomes the evidence that systems need to change.

What ties all of these definitions together is a common thread: action. Advocacy is not passive. It requires you to speak up, step forward, and use your voice. Whether that's literally telling your story, sitting at decision-making tables, fighting for policy changes, or making sure a patient gets the information they need to survive. The Pulse Center for Patient Safety Education and Advocacy puts it well: a patient advocate is a helper who helps the patient be more involved in their healthcare and hopefully receive better outcomes.

When I started as an ambassador with Fight CRC, I didn't realize that choosing awareness work versus research advocacy versus legislative advocacy were fundamentally different expressions of the same core commitment. I thought they were just different volunteer roles. But they weren't. Each one was advocacy. Each one was directed toward different leverage points in the system.

Why This Distinction Matters

You might be thinking: Tim, does this really matter? Isn't it all just helping people?

It matters immensely. Here's why.

When you understand yourself as an advocate rather than a volunteer, you operate from a place of expertise and authority. You're not grateful for the seat at the table. You know you belong there because you bring irreplaceable perspective. You're not hoping someone listens to your ideas. You're expecting they will, and you're prepared to push back when they don't. You're not supplementing an organization's work. You're fundamentally shaping it.

This matters for patients and families because advocacy creates real systemic change. It creates research that actually addresses patient needs. It creates policies that protect patients. It creates organizations that genuinely serve their communities instead of just talking about serving them.

It also matters for advocates themselves. Advocacy provides purpose and trajectory. It allows your patient experience to become your greatest professional asset rather than something you have to overcome or hide. It creates a career path, not just a volunteer role.

And it matters for organizations. Organizations that embed real advocacy into their DNA outperform those that don't. Not as a PR move, but as a fundamental operating principle. They make better decisions. They earn genuine trust from the communities they serve. They create sustainable impact.

I've saved over two dozen lives through my advocacy work. People heard me talk about screening and scheduled colonoscopies. Precancerous polyps were found and removed. Those people are alive today because I didn't stay silent. That's what advocacy can do. That's what real advocacy looks like.

A Quick Working Definition

All of these perspectives are right. That's the beautiful thing about advocacy. It's not a single rigid definition. It's a spectrum of ways people use their voice, experience, and energy to create change.

But for the purposes of this book, here's how I'm thinking about advocacy:

Advocacy is the act of using your voice, story, experience, and perspective to influence systems, decisions, and priorities in ways that benefit your community or cause. It requires you to show up authentically, stay informed, and be willing to speak up, even when it's uncomfortable.

Notice what's in there: your authentic voice, whether that's your patient story or professional expertise. And your willingness to actually shape outcomes. Notice what's not in there: the requirement for a fancy title, medical degree, or years of experience. You don't need any of those things to be an advocate.

What you do need is clarity about what you're advocating for and why it matters. You need to understand that there are different forms advocacy can take. Research advocacy. Legislative advocacy. Awareness advocacy. Fundraising advocacy. They all have value. And you need to recognize that choosing one path doesn't mean you're limited to it forever.

My journey took me from awareness to research to legislative work, and I'm still discovering new dimensions of what's possible. The common thread through all of it: I've been using my voice to create change. That's advocacy.

Wikipedia defines patient advocacy as a process in healthcare concerned with advocacy for patients, survivors, and caregivers, with typical activities including safeguarding patients from errors, protecting patient rights, awareness-building, and support and education. But I like to think about it more simply. Advocacy is when you refuse to accept things as they are and you take action to make them better. It's when your pain becomes your purpose.

Why You're Reading This

Whether you picked up this book because you're newly diagnosed and looking for direction, you've been volunteering for years and feel like something's missing, or you run an organization and want to embed real patient voices into your work, you're reading this because you sense there's something more.

There is. The 'something' is the healthcare advocate perspective.

Over the past few years, I've watched the healthcare advocacy land-scape evolve. Organizations that once treated patient input as a nice-to-have now recognize it as essential. Research institutions that once designed studies in isolation now actively partner with patients. Pharmaceutical companies that once saw patient advocates as a communication challenge now see them as strategic partners.

But this evolution is incomplete. There are still too many organizations with patient advisory boards that are purely performative. There are still researchers designing clinical trials without patient input from the start. There are still newly diagnosed patients who have no idea that their perspective is valuable to anyone beyond support groups.

This book exists to change that.

Throughout these pages, you'll learn what real advocacy looks like across different contexts. You'll understand the forms it takes. From research advocacy to legislative advocacy, fundraising advocacy and awareness advocacy. You'll learn how to move from personal experience to strategic influence. You'll discover how to build authentic patient engagement into organizations. And you'll understand how to measure whether your advocacy is actually creating the change you intend.

But more than anything, you'll learn how to find and articulate your why.

Because here's what I've learned: advocacy without a clear sense of purpose burns people out. Advocacy that's just about being busy or checking boxes becomes exhausting. But advocacy rooted in a deep understanding of what you're fighting for and why? That's sustainable. That's powerful. That's what creates real change.

Your Starting Point

Before we move forward, I want you to think about something.

What brought you to this book? What question are you asking? What gap are you feeling?

Maybe you're a newly diagnosed patient who wants to do more than just survive your diagnosis, to ensure others don't have to walk the same difficult path. Maybe you're a longtime volunteer who feels like you're doing important work, but you're hungry for something with more impact and influence. Maybe you're running an organization and genuinely want to serve your community, but you're not sure how to make patient voices a real part of your decision-making.

Whatever your starting point, know this: advocacy is a journey, not a destination. My journey took me from a scared cancer patient to someone who sits on national steering committees and mentors other advocates. That journey didn't happen overnight. It didn't happen because I'm special. It happened because I asked better questions and refused to accept surface-level engagement as good enough.

You can do the same. And that's what the rest of this book is about.

In the chapters ahead, we'll explore how the field of healthcare advocacy has evolved. We'll map the ecosystem you'll be operating within.

We'll dive into what patient advocacy actually looks like across different settings. And we'll give you the frameworks and tools to elevate your advocacy, whether you're just starting out or are ready to deepen the impact you're already creating.

But it all starts with understanding what advocacy really is. And recognizing that if you're reading this, you already know it's more than volunteering.

You're ready for something greater. Let's get started.

Chapter 2

The Evolution of Healthcare Advocacy as an Industry

Where It Started

Here's something that surprised me as I became more involved in advocacy. The patient advocacy movement didn't start with me. It didn't start five years ago when I was diagnosed. It started in the 1970s.

Back then, hospitals were opaque institutions (meaning patients had little visibility into how decisions were made or what their options were). Doctors and administrators controlled everything. Patients showed up, complied, and didn't ask many questions. The idea of a patient having a voice in their own care? That was radical.

But in the 1970s, something shifted. A growing patient rights movement started challenging this model. Advocates began pushing back against hospital paternalism. They demanded that patients have access to information. That patients have choices. That patients be treated as people, not just bodies to be fixed. This movement led to important milestones. The National Welfare Rights Organization's Patient Bill of Rights in 1970. The American Hospital Association's Patient Bill of Rights in 1972. These weren't just feel-good documents. They formalized the idea that patients had rights that needed to be protected.

But here's the thing about those early days of advocacy. It was mostly happening in hospitals. It was mostly about protecting people from bad things going wrong. It was defensive. It was necessary, but it was limited.

The field I've witnessed evolve over the past five to ten years is fundamentally different from that. And understanding how that shift happened matters if you're going to understand where advocacy is heading.

The Technology Shift

When I started my community management career, we didn't have the tools we have today—not just social media, but also data analytics, CRM systems, and dedicated community platforms. There was no analytics dashboard showing me exactly how many people engaged with a post. There was no way to segment communities or identify the most active members. We were making educated guesses. We were engaged in a lot of manual work. We were being pretty informal about it.

Then social media evolved.

The early 2010s saw healthcare organizations starting to explore Face-book, Twitter, and blogs. Mayo Clinic became an early leader in this space. In 2010, they established the Social Media Health Network to provide what they called an "authentic voice for patients and health care professionals, building relationships through the revolutionary power of social media." But here's what was interesting about those early days. A lot of organizations treated social media as a distribution channel. They posted information. People could see it. Maybe they'd comment. But it wasn't really dialogue. It was still mostly one-way communication.

I remember when I first became involved with community management. We'd post something and hope people would engage. We didn't have the tools to know who was really involved, what they cared about, or how to build real relationships with them. We were using Twitter and Facebook the same way we'd use a megaphone. We were broadcasting, not building community.

Over the past few years, something shifted. Instead of trying to manage communities on platforms that social media companies own, organizations started building dedicated platforms. Community platforms they actually control. Where the rules are clearer. Where people know they're joining a community specifically for that health condition or organization. These platforms give us the data we need. They give us the tools to have actual conversations. They help us understand who our advocates are and what they need.

This shift from social media to dedicated community platforms is massive. It represents a move from broadcast to conversation. From "here's information we think you need" to "here's where we listen to what you need."

The Regulatory Wake-Up Call

Around the same time social media was expanding, something else was happening in Washington.

The Patient Protection and Affordable Care Act, passed in 2010, did something that fundamentally changed the healthcare research land-scape. It created the Patient-Centered Outcomes Research Institute (PCORI)—a nonprofit organization funded by Congress to improve the quality and relevance of healthcare research by involving patients as partners.

This wasn't just another funding mechanism. This was Congress saying something pretty radical: if you want federal funding for comparative effectiveness research, you must involve patients in the research. Not as subjects. As partners.

Think about that for a second. Before PCORI, research was designed by researchers. Researchers decided what questions were worth asking. They decided what outcomes mattered. Patients showed up to participate. But patients didn't actually shape the research.

PCORI required something different. They required meaningful engagement of patients in the research process. Patients needed to be involved in determining study design. In selecting what outcomes the research would measure. In interpreting the results.

In 2011, PCORI commissioned systematic reviews to figure out how to effectively engage patients in research. They developed something called the PCORI Engagement Rubric. This wasn't just a nice-to-have, but a requirement. If researchers wanted PCORI funding, they needed to follow this rubric. They needed to show how they were engaging patients as true partners.

This was a regulatory mandate. And it fundamentally changed who had a seat at the health research table.

As someone who,   last year, started serving as a CDMRP peer reviewer, I saw this firsthand. I wasn't there because someone was being nice to me, but because federal funding requirements said I needed to be there. My perspective mattered because Congress said it mattered.

That doesn't mean engagement is always done well. Some organizations still treat patient engagement like a compliance box to check. But the mandate exists. The requirement exists. And that changed everything.

The Evidence Solidified

But the real reason advocacy isn't going away is because the evidence keeps showing the same thing: patients who are engaged in their care have better outcomes.

This isn't my opinion. This is what the research shows.

In 2013, Health Affairs published a systematic review looking at the evidence on patient engagement.[1] They found that patients who participate in their healthcare decisions report higher levels of satisfaction. They have more knowledge about their conditions and treatments. They're more likely to stick with treatment plans. And in some cases, they actually have improved health outcomes.

The CDC has documented this as well, finding an association between higher patient activation and improved health outcomes, as well as lower costs two years later.[2]

When PCORI published early findings on the impact of patient engagement in research, they found something consistent across the studies. Patient engagement provided valuable contributions to research feasibility, improving acceptability and research rigor. It also made the research more relevant to the people it was supposed to help.

These aren't marginal improvements. This is significant evidence that the way research is undertaken matters. And that who is involved in designing research matters.

So, when healthcare organizations started thinking about embedding patient engagement into their work, they weren't acting just because it felt right. They were responding because the evidence showed it worked.

My Own Evolution Mirrors the Field's

I want to tie this back to my own journey because I think it illustrates what's been happening at scale across the healthcare system.

When I started working in community management seventeen years ago, we were handling basic things. Building email lists. Creating Facebook pages. Starting blogs. It was informal. We didn't have many systems or processes as we were figuring things out as we went.

As I progressed in community management, we built better tools. We started tracking metrics. Understanding data. Building intentional strategies instead of just hoping engagement would happen. But it was still mostly about awareness. About getting information out to as many people as we could reach.

Then, at the age of 52, I was diagnosed with cancer and became part of the community I was serving. And everything I thought I knew about community management suddenly felt incomplete.

When I started with Fight CRC as an ambassador, I quickly realized there were other ways to be involved. Research advocacy. Legislative advocacy. Fundraising. Awareness. I gravitated toward awareness because that was my experience over seventeen years. But over time, I explored the other areas. And I realized something: the infrastructure that exists for patient advocacy now didn't exist before. The platforms. The funding. The regulatory requirements. The evidence base.

None of that was in place when I started my community management career. It was all created in the last decade.

I went from being a community manager who happened to be a patient, to being a patient who could actually shape research. Who could sit on steering committees. Who could influence policy. Who could mentor other advocates. That progression I experienced isn't unique. That's the trajectory of the entire field.

What This Means

Here's what I think is important about understanding this evolution. The shift from the 1970s patient rights movement to what we're seeing today isn't just a difference in scale. It's a difference in where patients are seated.

From Patient to Advocate

In the 1970s and 1980s, patient advocates fought for a seat at the table. We need to be heard, they said.

In the 1990s and 2000s, patient advocates started winning seats, but they were often the seats someone else decided to give them.

Now? Now, there are regulatory requirements that patients must be at the table. There's evidence that shows it improves outcomes. There's funding that supports patient engagement. And there are dedicated platforms and tools that make it easier to engage patients meaningfully instead of performatively.

Organizations that now embed real patient engagement into their DNA are outperforming those that don't. They're making better decisions. They're earning genuine trust from the communities they serve. They're creating more sustainable impact.

But here's the thing. And I want to be honest about this. This evolution isn't complete. There are still plenty of organizations with patient advisory boards that are purely performative. There are still researchers designing studies without talking to patients. There are still patients with no idea their perspective is valuable.

The infrastructure for authentic patient advocacy has been built. The evidence supports it. The regulatory requirements demand it. But the cultural shift? That's still happening. And that's where real advocates come in.

Because advocacy isn't just about having a seat at the table. It's about making sure that seat actually changes what happens at the table.

That's the evolution I've witnessed. And I think understanding it helps you understand where advocacy is heading.

Chapter 3

The Advocacy Ecosystem
and Its Forms

Not All Advocacy Looks the Same

One of the most important things I learned during my first year as an advocate is that there are many different ways to show up. When I became an ambassador with Fight CRC, I thought advocacy was mostly about raising awareness. Telling my story. Educating people about colorectal cancer screening. That felt right to me. It felt aligned with my skill set. And it was valuable work.

But then I started exploring the other areas. I attended legislative events. I participated in research committees. I watched how fundraising worked. And I realized something crucial: advocacy isn't monolithic. There are multiple forms. Multiple entry points. Multiple ways to make real change happen. And just as importantly, different people are drawn to different forms based on their skills, energy, and what fills their cup.

This diversity is one of the most beautiful things about the advocacy ecosystem. You don't have to be all things. You can find your place. You can contribute in the way that makes sense for you.

The Four Forms of Advocacy

Let me map out what I'm talking about. There are four distinct forms of advocacy operating in healthcare right now. They're interconnected. They often support each other. But they're distinct enough that under-standing the differences matters.

Awareness Advocacy

Awareness advocacy is about visibility. It's about making sure people know a disease exists. That they know how to recognize symptoms. That they know screening or prevention is possible. That they under-stand the impact the disease has on patients and families.

Awareness advocacy looks like Fight CRC's #StrongArmSelfie campaign, where people post photos using the hashtag and funds go directly to research. It looks like their United in Blue installation on the national mall, with over 27,000 blue flags representing people under 50 projected to be diagnosed with colorectal cancer by 2030. It's powerful because it makes the invisible visible.

Awareness advocacy also looks like storytelling. Like my story being featured in publications so other patients see themselves reflected back. It's educational content. Webinars. Podcasts. Social media campaigns. Community events. Basically, any effort to help people understand a disease or condition exists and that something can be done about it.

Man Up to Cancer engages in significant awareness work, and their entire model is built on making men feel less alone in their cancer journey. They host in-person gatherings and online communities. They produce a podcast. They help men understand that reaching out for help isn't weakness. That's awareness advocacy at work, changing how people perceive cancer and masculinity.

The beautiful thing about awareness advocacy is that it doesn't require a medical degree. You don't need to understand clinical trial design.

You just need to be willing to share your story and help people under-stand why it matters.

Research Advocacy

Research advocacy is about ensuring patient voices shape the research that gets done and how it gets done. It's not just about raising aware-ness so people want to participate in research, but sitting at the table where research priorities get decided. Where research gets designed. Where outcomes get selected.

Fight CRC runs their Research Advocacy Training and Support program, which they call RATS, training advocates to become educated patient voices on research committees. These advocates sit on advisory boards, steering committees, and helping researchers under-stand what matters to patients so research gets designed around their needs rather than just scientific curiosity.

When I started serving as a CDMRP peer reviewer, I was engaged in research advocacy, reviewing research grant applications and providing patient perspective on whether the proposed research would actually address something patients cared about. I was on steering committees for trials, helping shape how the research unfolded.

Research advocacy also happens through patient advisory boards at pharmaceutical companies, academic research centers, and diagnostic companies. It happens on institutional review boards, in meetings where patients help interpret research results so they can be translated into language patients actually understand.

HOPA, the Hematology/Oncology Pharmacy Association, engages in research advocacy by working with researchers and pharmaceutical companies to ensure patient perspectives inform how medications are developed, tested, and ultimately delivered to patients. They have patient advisory panels and outreach committees specifically designed to amplify patient voices in research.

Research advocacy requires a willingness to learn. You might not understand everything about clinical trial methodology when you start; instead, you contribute your deep expertise in lived experience. That's what matters. That's what the research world needs.

Legislative Advocacy

Legislative advocacy is about getting policies changed. Laws passed. Regulations reformed. It's about walking into legislator offices and saying: here's what my community needs. Here's what needs to change in policy to make that happen.

Fight CRC engages in significant legislative advocacy through their Call-on Congress event every year in March. They bring advocates to Washington to meet with their elected officials and push for policy change, and have successfully lobbied for multiple victories: lowering the colorectal cancer screening age from 50 to 45, and removing out-of-pocket costs for colonoscopies. Their Catalyst State-by-State Advocacy Program funds grassroots legislative efforts in states across the country, and has helped pass legislation in Kentucky, Arkansas, Rhode Island, and Texas, all focused on removing barriers to screening.

PAN Foundation performs legislative advocacy around healthcare affordability and access. They bring patients to Capitol Hill through their Advocacy Action Summit, educating lawmakers about problems like copay accumulator policies that prevent patients from using assistance to pay for medications. They advocate for policies that make healthcare more accessible and affordable.

Legislative advocacy is about power. It's about understanding how systems work and leveraging that understanding to change them. When I started with legislative work, I was intimidated, thinking one had to be an expert. That you had to understand healthcare policy inside and out. But what I learned is that legislators want to hear from their constituents. They want to understand the real impact of policies on real people. Your story matters. Your presence matters.

The beautiful thing about legislative advocacy is that it doesn't have to be huge. You don't have to go to Washington. You can simply contact your state representative. You can testify at a local hearing. You can call your congressperson. Legislative advocacy happens at every level.

Fundraising Advocacy

Fundraising advocacy is about mobilizing resources. Money. It's about asking people to contribute financially to support the cause. Some of that might be grassroots fundraising, where individuals ask friends and family. Some might be major donor cultivation, where you build relationships with wealthy individuals or corporations. Others might be corporate sponsorships or partnerships.

Fight CRC raises funds for their research grants. Their Lisa Fund has awarded over 350,000 dollars to support research on advanced colorectal cancer. That money doesn't come from nowhere. It comes from fundraising advocacy. From people asking others to give.

Man Up to Cancer supports their mission partly through fundraising. They host events. They ask for donations. The Gathering of Wolves retreat they host each year requires fundraising to take place.

PAN Foundation raises funds through individual donations and corporate partnerships. Since their founding, they've given over 4 billion dollars in financial assistance to patients. That kind of impact requires serious fundraising.

Here's where I want to be honest about my own relationship with fundraising advocacy. I discovered pretty quickly that repeated fundraising asks didn't feel right to me. I'd spent years grassroots fundraising and had built significant relationships with my professional network. When I started my advocacy work, I realized I'd already asked those relationships for a lot. I didn't want to keep asking for money over and over, so I made a choice.

Fundraising advocacy isn't my lane.

That doesn't mean it's not important. It is. Advocacy needs funding. Research needs funding. Programs need funding. But it also doesn't mean everyone has to do it. The beautiful thing about the advocacy ecosystem is that you get to choose.

Who's Involved

The organizations involved with advocacy work look different depending on the form of advocacy. And a lot of organizations under-take multiple forms.

Nonprofits like Fight CRC and PAN Foundation operate across multiple forms, engaging in awareness work, research advocacy, legislative advocacy, and some also fundraise.

Patient support organizations like Man Up to Cancer conducts aware-ness work and fundraising, and they often do light legislative work when it affects their community.

Over the past decade, pharmaceutical companies and diagnostics firms have become more sophisticated about patient engagement. Companies like Exact Sciences engage with patients through advisory boards and research partnerships–research advocacy–which means they're less likely to be involved in legislative advocacy (though that's changing). They're definitely involved in awareness because it's good for their business when more people get screened for colorectal cancer.

Research institutions like hospitals and academic medical centers have patient advisory boards and research partnerships. They engage in research advocacy because they have to. PCORI requires it, but many are doing it authentically now.

Government agencies fund research. The National Cancer Institute partners with patient advocates, and NIH is increasingly requiring patient engagement.

There are also professional associations like HOPA, which brings together pharmacy professionals and, increasingly, patient voices.

HOPA has a Patient Outreach Committee and engages in both research and legislative advocacy.

The point is that the ecosystem is diverse, with many types of organizations involved, many entry points, and many ways to be part of creating change.

How They Intersect

Here's where it gets really interesting. The following four forms of advocacy don't exist in silos. They actually support each other.

Awareness advocacy creates the foundation. When you raise awareness about colorectal cancer screening, more people get screened. More people get diagnosed early. More people survive. That creates a larger patient community. A community of people with stakes in the outcomes. That gives legislative advocates a larger group to mobilize. You can't pass legislation if you don't have people who care about that legislation.

Research advocacy informs legislative advocacy. When research shows that patients want personalized treatment options, but the regulatory system doesn't allow for certain innovations, legislative advocates can point to that research and say: here's what we need to change. When research shows that screening saves lives, legislative advocates use that data to push for policies that increase access to screening.

Fundraising advocacy supports everything else. Research advocacy doesn't happen without funding for research. Awareness campaigns don't happen without funding for campaigns. Legislative advocacy sometimes doesn't happen without funding to bring advocates to the capitol.

And awareness advocacy is strengthened by legislative wins and research breakthroughs. When you can say, "look, this policy changed and now more people have access to screening," that makes your awareness message stronger. When you can say, "look, this research discovery means new treatment options," that builds hope and momentum.

My own journey illustrates this. I started with awareness advocacy because that was familiar to me. Then I explored research advocacy because I realized I didn't need a science background; I just needed to listen carefully and advocate for patients. Then I explored legislative work and discovered it filled my soul. I intentionally didn't conduct fundraising because that wasn't aligned with my values. But each form I've engaged in has strengthened the others. Sharing my story (aware-ness) gave me credibility in research spaces, and understanding research challenges informed what I could advocate for legislatively.

Finding Your Form

Here's what I want to emphasize because it matters: you don't have to do everything, you don't have to be equally skilled at all four forms, and you don't have to like all four forms. The beauty of this ecosystem is that it needs all four. And different people are drawn to different forms.

Some people are natural storytellers. They should do awareness advocacy.

Some people love diving into detail and want to understand research. They should do research advocacy.

Some people love politics, power dynamics, and want to influence policy. They should do legislative advocacy.

Some people are skilled at relationship-building and fundraising. They should do fundraising advocacy.

Most importantly, you get to choose what fills your cup. What feels aligned with who you are. What you have energy for. Not everyone is a fundraiser. Not everyone is a researcher. Not everyone is a lobbyist. Not everyone is a storyteller. But everyone has something to contribute.

The advocacy ecosystem works because we have different people doing different things. I do awareness, research, and legislative advocacy. I don't repeatedly engage with fundraising. That's fine. Someone else loves fundraising and isn't interested in legislative work. That's fine too. We need both.

So, when you're thinking about how you want to be involved in advocacy, ask yourself this: What form speaks to me? What feels like work I could do? What would make me feel like I'm actually creating change? The answers to those questions will point you toward your place in the ecosystem. And that place matters. Because this work only happens when all the different pieces come together. And that only happens when people show up in the ways that are authentic to them.

The Ecosystem Is Growing

One last thing I want to note: the ecosystem I'm describing is relatively new in its current form. Five years ago, most of it didn't exist the way it does now. There wasn't formal research advocacy training for patients. There wasn't the same funding for legislative advocacy by patients. There wasn't the same recognition that pharmaceutical companies should engage with patients in research.

But that's changing. Fast. More organizations are adding patient advisory boards. More funding is requiring patient engagement. More research is being designed with patients at the table from the beginning. The ecosystem is becoming more mature. More sophisticated. More inclusive.

Which means opportunities are growing. If you're interested in advocacy, there's likely a place for you. A form that fits. An organization that needs your voice. An opportunity to be part of this work.

That's the ecosystem. That's how it works. And that's where real change happens.

Chapter 4

Starting Your Advocacy Journey

The Days Right After

I remember the moment I got home after being told I had cancer. It was a few days after diagnosis. I was sitting in my house, and the weight of it all was settling in. Stage IV colorectal cancer. Metastatic to the liver. Treatment ahead. Uncertainty about my future.

And then something shifted. I remember thinking: there has to be a reason this is happening. I've always believed that everything happens for a reason. But that belief wasn't comforting in a passive way. It wasn't about accepting what happened and being okay with it. It was about figuring out what I was supposed to do with it. What was my role in this?

And then the answer came to me, clear and simple. My reason was to make sure nobody else I knew would have to go through what I was about to go through. To do whatever I could to prevent others from having this experience. Or to help them navigate it if they did.

That purpose became my anchor. In the days and weeks that followed, when the fear and the overwhelming weight of diagnosis threatened to take over, I could come back to that. I have a reason for this. I have something I'm supposed to do with this.

For many people, that's where advocacy begins. Not in a strategic planning session. Not in a board meeting. It begins in those raw early days after diagnosis when you're trying to make sense of what's happening to you. When you're looking for some kind of meaning or purpose in something that feels completely senseless.

If you're in those early days right now, I want you to know something. That search for meaning isn't weakness. It's not denial. It's one of the most human things we do. And if it points you toward advocacy, toward wanting to help others, that's not something to dismiss. That's something to follow.

Finding Your People

But here's the thing about that initial purpose: it doesn't happen in isolation. You can't do this alone. The first real step in starting your advocacy journey isn't figuring out which form of advocacy to do. It's finding your people. Finding others who understand what you're going through because they're going through it too.

For me, that started in an unexpected way. A friend of mine, who doesn't have cancer, suggested I join Man Up to Cancer. I was surprised by the suggestion. I'm not a man. But I took a look at what they were doing. I saw their Wolfpack community. I saw they were focused on building connection and understanding for people dealing with cancer. And I joined.

At first, I was intimidated. I was newly diagnosed. I didn't feel like I had anything to contribute. But I showed up anyway. And I found something I desperately needed. I found people who got me. Who understood what it felt like to receive a diagnosis like mine. Who weren't going to tell me to stay positive or be strong. Who just got it.

From there, I found COLONTOWN, an online community specifically for people dealing with colorectal cancer, particularly those with metastatic disease. I found treatment options there. I found people further along in their journey who could answer questions I didn't even know how to ask. I found hope in their stories.

Then I applied to become an ambassador with Fight CRC. And that opened another door. Another community. Another set of people who were living this experience.

I say this because I want you to understand something. You probably won't find your people by accident. You have to be willing to look. You have to be willing to put yourself out there. You have to be willing to share what you're going through.

When I announced my diagnosis, I was overwhelmed with information. People sent me articles, treatment recommendations, and advice. It was too much. But then a former co-worker introduced me to her uncle, Chuck, who had stage IV colon cancer. He wasn't on social media, so she gave him my number and he called me.

And something shifted. Chuck wasn't sending me information from the internet. He was sharing his actual lived experience. He was telling me what he'd been through. What he wished he'd known. And because he had actually lived through it, I could believe him in a way I couldn't believe the information coming at me from everywhere else.

Chuck became my first real connection in this journey. Not because I sought him out strategically. But because I was open to the connection when it came.

That's the first real step. Being willing to be open. Being willing to share what's happening to you. Being willing to say: I need help. I need to talk to someone who understands.

Online and In-Person

Once you start opening up, you'll probably find communities. Online communities like MUTC and COLONTOWN were lifelines for me, especially in those early pandemic days when in-person connections weren't always possible. They provided 24/7 connection. Someone was always awake. Someone was always dealing with something simi-lar. You could post your question at 3 a.m. and get responses from people who understood.

But here's something I learned that I think is important: online communities are amazing. In the early days, they saved me. But they're not the whole picture.

I met Lee Silverstein through a MUTC Wolfpack meetup on Zoom. We talked online for a while, and then we realized we were both being treated at the same cancer center. We soon started coordinating our infusions, seeing each other there in person, and then something shifted.

When you're sitting next to someone in an infusion chair, both of you going through treatment, something human happens that can't happen online. You can see each other. You can offer a hand when someone's having a hard time. You can share a laugh about something only someone going through the same thing would find funny. You can ask follow-up questions. You can have a conversation that's not mediated by a screen.

I learned that in-person connections provide something online connections can't replicate. They give you the chance to really know some-one, to see their humanity, and to build real relationships.

So if you're starting your advocacy journey, my advice is this: start where you can. Online communities are valuable. Especially when you're newly diagnosed and maybe not ready to share your face or voice with other people. But also look for in-person opportunities when you're ready. Attend support group meetings. Go to retreats. Show up at events. The human touch matters more than you might think.

And don't underestimate the power of one-on-one conversation. The phone call with Chuck. The in-person infusion meetings with Lee. These are where real connection happens. This is where you start to understand that you're not alone. This is where you start to see that other people have navigated this and survived. And thrived.

The Weight of Loss

But I need to be honest about something that doesn't get talked about enough in advocacy spaces. The more people you come into contact with, the more relationships you build, the more people you advocate alongside, the more loss you experience. And it gets harder.

Chuck passed away from cancer. Lee passed away from cancer. The more time I spend in this space, the more people I meet, the more people I build relationships with, the more I lose. And every single loss hits.

When you're newly diagnosed, you meet people further along in their journey. You think: okay, they're doing well, they've survived, there's hope. And then one day you learn they've passed. You realize that surviving the initial diagnosis doesn't mean surviving long-term. You realize that the person you were just talking to, the person whose advice helped you, the person whose story gave you hope, is gone.

It's devastating. And it's part of this work.

I want to be clear about something. I'm not saying this to discourage you from starting your advocacy journey. I'm saying it because you deserve to know what you're getting into. You deserve to understand that the relationships you build in this space are real and precious and also fragile. You deserve to know that the cost of doing this work is grief.

But here's what I've learned. If I want to be angry at cancer for taking Chuck and Lee, I need to also acknowledge that cancer is what brought them into my life in the first place. And I don't want to do that. I don't want to regret knowing them. I don't want to regret the conversations we shared. I don't want to regret the ways they shaped my advocacy and my life.

So instead of letting the grief paralyze me, I try to channel it. I let it fuel my advocacy work. I let it remind me why this matters. Every person I lose makes me more committed to making sure others don't have to go through what they went through. It makes me more committed to finding cures. To changing systems. To saving lives.

The loss is real. The grief is real. But so is the meaning we can make from it. And the relationships we build in this space, even the ones that end in loss, are worth it.

This is something to prepare yourself for as you enter this space. You will likely lose people. You will grieve. That's not a reason to stay away. That's a reason to go in with eyes open. To know that you're building something real with real people facing real mortality. And to let that reality sharpen your sense of purpose.

Sharing Your Story

Here's something that happened gradually for me, and I think it's important to acknowledge. The more I shared my story one-on-one with someone else, the easier it became to share it publicly with strangers.

When I first shared my diagnosis, it was hard. It felt vulnerable. It felt like I was admitting something shameful. But as I told my story to Chuck, and then to Lee, and then to others in the community, some-thing changed. The story stopped feeling like a secret. It stopped feeling like something that defined me negatively. It became just my story. A thing that happened. Something I was navigating.

And then telling it became easier. Sharing it in support groups. Sharing it at events. Speaking about it publicly. Because I'd already told it so many times, to so many people, in so many different ways, that by the time I was telling it to a room full of strangers, it didn't feel foreign anymore.

If you're in the early days of your advocacy journey, and you're not ready to share your story publicly yet, that's fine. Start small. Tell one trusted person. Then tell another. Build your comfort level gradually. Because one of the most powerful tools in advocacy is your story. And you don't have to be ready to share it publicly right away. You can build up to that.

But I also want to say this: your story matters. Not because it's perfect or inspiring or follows some particular arc. It matters because it's yours. Because it's real. Because when you share it, someone else hears it and thinks: oh my God, I'm not the only one. That person feels less alone. That's advocacy. That's powerful.

Finding Your Form

As you start connecting with people, you'll probably start noticing the different ways they're involved. You'll see people doing awareness work. People doing research work. People doing legislative work. People doing fundraising.

If you remember from Chapter 3, there are four main forms of advocacy: awareness, research, legislative, and fundraising. They all matter. They all create change. And you don't have to do all of them.

When I started, I gravitated toward awareness because that's what felt familiar. I knew how to tell stories. I knew how to build community. Awareness work felt natural to me. So I leaned into that.

But as I became more comfortable, I explored the other forms and discovered I had something to offer in research spaces. I discovered I had passion for legislative work and that I didn't want to carry out repeated fundraising tasks.

You might be the opposite. You might hate the spotlight and love the details of research. You might be natural at building relationships with donors. You might be passionate about policy.

The beautiful thing is you get to choose. You get to try different things and see what fits. You get to contribute in the way that feels right to you.

But here's the thing: you can't figure out what fits until you get involved. Until you show up. Until you try.

The Emotional Reality

I need to be honest about something. Starting your advocacy journey while you're dealing with a serious diagnosis is hard. It's really hard.

You're dealing with treatment, fear, the practical reality of navigating the medical system, grief over the life you thought you were going to lead, and the unknown.

And now you're also trying to show up for others. Trying to share your story. Trying to learn. Trying to contribute.

It's a lot.

I had an advantage that I want to acknowledge. I've been practicing mindfulness, consciousness, and meditation for about a decade before my diagnosis. That practice helped in ways I can't overstate. My diagnosis was a fact. It helped me understand that I couldn't change what happened. But I could change how I reacted to it. I could choose where I put my energy. I could choose to focus on what I could control rather than spiraling about what I couldn't.

That practice doesn't make the difficulty disappear. It just makes it more manageable.

If you don't have that practice, I'm not saying you need to take it up right now. You have enough on your plate. But I am saying this: take care of your mental health. If you need a therapist, get one. If you need to take a break from advocacy to focus on your treatment, do that. If you need to step back from your advocacy work for a few weeks or months, that's not failure. That's taking care of yourself.

There's nothing wrong with needing help. There's nothing wrong with not being able to do it all. There's nothing wrong with admitting you're overwhelmed.

In fact, I think there's something really healthy about admitting that. Because advocacy that burns you out isn't sustainable. Advocacy that costs your mental health isn't the kind of advocacy we need.

It Gets Easier

I think about starting advocacy like starting a fitness routine. If you've never worked out before, the first time you visit the gym, your body is sore. Everything hurts. You're out of breath. You wonder why anyone would voluntarily do this.

But if you stick with it, something changes. Your body adapts. The exercises get easier. And then something remarkable happens. You start feeling better than you ever have in your life. You have more energy. You feel stronger. You feel capable.

For me, advocacy is like that. Those early days when I was learning how to share my story, learning how to engage with online communities, learning how to show up for others while I was terrified about my own future, those were hard. It was like those first gym sessions. Everything felt difficult.

But I stuck with it. And it got easier. The fear didn't go away, but it became something I could hold alongside the purpose. The difficulty didn't disappear, but I developed capacity I didn't know I had.

And now when I take on something new in advocacy, like joining HOPA's Patient Advisory Panel, or starting a research review, I still feel that initial soreness. That initial overwhelm. But I know from experience that if I stick with it, I'll come through the other side. I'll develop new skills. I'll build new relationships. I'll find new ways to contribute.

And I'll feel stronger for it.

Your First Steps

So if you're just starting your advocacy journey, here's what I'd encourage you to do.

First, find your people. Look for an online community related to your diagnosis. Join a support group. Reach out to someone you know who's been through something similar. Be willing to share what you're going through. Be willing to be vulnerable.

Second, start small. You don't have to speak at a conference, serve on a board, or do anything public right away. Share your story with one person. Then another. Build your comfort level gradually.

Third, explore. Pay attention to the different ways people are contributing. See what resonates with you. What excites you. What makes you feel like you're creating change in a way that feels authentic to you.

Fourth, take care of yourself. Your mental health matters more than your productivity in advocacy. It's okay to slow down. It's okay to ask for help. It's okay to take a break.

And finally, remember why you're doing this. Whether your why is the same as mine, or different, hold onto it. Because that why is what will sustain you when things get hard. That why is what will keep you going.

The advocacy journey isn't easy. But it's one of the most meaningful things you can do with your experience. And you don't have to do it alone. There are people out there, right now, going through exactly what you're going through. Communities waiting for you. Mentors who have been where you are.

You just have to be willing to show up. To be vulnerable. To share your story. And to let others do the same.

That's where it starts. That's where it begins.

Chapter 5

From Personal Experience
to Strategic Voice

The Unexpected Moment

I remember the first time I was offered money for my time as a patient, $150 for an hour. A company wanted my perspective on something, calling it patient research. I thought: great, easy money. I'm in.

I didn't realize at the time that I was doing research advocacy. I didn't have some grand vision of becoming a patient expert. I was just being honest. Sharing my thoughts and experiences. It seemed simple because it was simple. They asked me questions. I answered them. Honest answers based on what I'd actually lived through.

Those opportunities started multiplying. One survey led to another. A different organization wanted to talk to me. Then another. I kept saying yes because each one was easy and helped me understand that my perspective had value beyond just my own situation.

Then I was asked to serve on a steering committee, to participate in research design, not just provide feedback on existing research, to be a peer reviewer for CDMRP grant applications, and actually help shape the research that would be conducted.

That was different. That was when I realized I had moved from just sharing my story to actually wielding influence over research priorities and design. That was when I felt like I'd been elevated to a different level of advocacy.

But here's the thing: there wasn't one defining moment where I trans-formed from patient to expert. Looking back, I can see the evolution clearly. But in the moment, I was just showing up. Just being honest. Just saying yes to opportunities that came my way.

Know Your Audience

The most important thing I learned about transforming personal experience into strategic voice is this: it's not about choosing between story and expertise. It's about understanding who you're talking to and what they actually need from you.

When I talk to someone recently diagnosed, my story is the most important thing I can offer. They don't need my data. They need to know that someone has walked this path and survived. They need to hear that it's possible to keep going. They need the human element. The hope. The lived experience.

When I talk to my oncologist about pursuing a liver transplant, I can't lead with just my story. My oncologist has heard thousands of patient stories. What I need is to combine my story with data. I need to say: here's what I've learned through my experience. Here's what the research shows. Here's what I need from you. That combination is what moves him to action.

When I talk to a legislative aide about policy change, I lead with my personal story because it makes the policy real. It makes it human. But I back it up with data. I say: I experienced this problem because of this policy. Here's how many other patients are experiencing it. Here's the research that shows what needs to change. Here's the solution. Story plus data equals persuasion.

When I talk with my friends who aren't thinking about cancer at all, who believe it will never happen to them, my story is critical. I'm not trying to convince them of policy or research priority. I'm trying to get them to understand that this can happen. That screening matters. That early detection saves lives. My story is the vehicle for that message.

The key is understanding your audience. What do they already know? What are they skeptical about? What will actually change their minds or move them to action? Once you understand that, you can calibrate your approach.

Sometimes that's pure story. Sometimes that's pure data. Most often, it's a combination. But the combination is intentional. It's tailored to who you're talking to.

Your Story Is Your Authority

Let me be very clear about something because I think it matters. Nobody knows your story like you do. Nobody has a right to challenge you on your experience. Nobody has the authority to tell you that your story isn't valid.

But here's the flip side: if you're timid about sharing it, if you seem nervous or uncertain, people will pick up on that. And uncertainty sounds like you're not sure about what you're saying. It sounds like maybe you don't fully trust your own experience.

The antidote to that is confidence. Not arrogance. Not pretending you know more than you do. But confidence in your own story. Confidence that what you experienced is real. Confidence that your perspective matters.

I learned this because I had to learn it. In the early days, I wasn't confident about my story. I felt like maybe I should apologize for taking up space. Like maybe other people's stories were more important. Like maybe being stage IV made my story more valuable than someone at stage II, and how could I presume to speak if I was only stage II?

But then I realized something. The person at stage II who gets early detection and survives has a different story than I do. It's not less important. It's not less valuable. It's just different. Their story might connect with someone else's experience in a way mine never could.

I relate to white males in their 50s or 60s with grown kids, a wife, living in the suburbs. But my story might not connect with someone who's Filipino, living in a rural area, in their 30s with young kids and a wife. That person needs to hear from someone who shares their context. Someone whose story they can see themselves in.

This is why diversity of voices in advocacy matters. This is why your story matters even if it's not the most severe diagnosis or the most dramatic journey. Your story matters because someone needs to hear it. Someone needs to feel less alone because you had the courage to share.

So when you're transforming your personal experience into strategic voice, start with this: believe in your story. Trust your experience, and speak with confidence about what you've actually lived through. Because nobody can argue with that. Nobody can tell you that you didn't experience what you experienced.

From Volunteer to Expert

For me, the real shift from feeling like a volunteer to feeling like an expert patient happened gradually. I was doing the work. Showing up. Being active in the organizations I joined. Saying yes to opportunities. Being consistent.

And then, one day, a fellow advocate reached out to me, asking how I'd navigated something related to my treatment. They said they'd heard about my experience and wondered if I could help them think through their options. They were asking me for my expertise.

That was the moment. Not because some official title changed. Not because I got certified in something. But because someone who was also living this experience was coming to me and treating my knowledge as valuable. They were acknowledging that I'd learned something through my journey that could help them.

That's when I felt like I'd crossed from volunteering into expertise. When fellow advocates started coming to me. When organizations started asking me to serve on committees not just as a voice, but as someone who could help shape decisions. When people recognized that I'd accumulated knowledge and experience that was worth their time to access.

But I want to be clear about how that happened. It wasn't because I was special. It wasn't because I had a medical degree or fancy credential. It was because I kept showing up. I kept being honest. I kept engaging with the work. I kept sharing what I'd learned.

I also want to name something else. Early in my advocacy journey, someone asked how I'd gotten in touch with my transplant team, telling me their oncologist hadn't mentioned that a liver transplant was an option. They wanted to know what my oncologist had done.

And I had to tell them the truth: my oncologist didn't mention it. I pursued it. I researched it. I found the program. I told him I wanted to pursue it. He didn't hand it to me on a platter. I had to advocate for myself to even start the conversation.

That's when I realized something important. My expertise wasn't just in my experience as a patient. It was in my advocacy for myself. In my willingness to question what doctors told me. In my refusal to accept the first opinion as the final answer. In my proactive approach to my own care.

When I shared that with someone else, I wasn't just sharing my story. I was sharing a strategy. A way of approaching their own healthcare. That's when patient experience becomes patient expertise. When you can translate what you've learned into something actionable for someone else.

Earning Credibility

Credibility as a patient expert isn't earned through credentials or time spent in medical school. It's earned through consistency, showing up, and being active in the work over time.

You get out what you put in. That's simple, but it's true. If you say yes to opportunities and then disappear, you don't build credibility. If you show up to one meeting and then ghost the organization, you don't build credibility. But if you keep saying yes. If you keep showing up. If you keep being active. If you keep sharing your story. Over time, people recognize you as someone they can rely on. Someone whose perspective they value. Someone who's invested in this work.

I didn't plan this. I didn't set out to build credibility as a patient expert. I just kept saying yes. To the surveys. To the committees. To the peer review. To the speaking opportunities. To the mentoring. And, over time, a reputation emerged. People started knowing who I was. Started asking for my input. Started treating me as an expert.

The other thing I realized is that expertise comes from depth of engagement with one area. I'm not an expert in everything. I'm not equally knowledgeable about all forms of cancer or all treatment options. But I am deeply knowledgeable about colorectal cancer. About metastatic disease. About the liver transplant option. About what it takes to be a patient advocate. About how to navigate the research and legislative spaces.

That deep knowledge, combined with willingness to say I don't know about other areas, is what builds credibility. You're not pretending to be an expert in everything. You're being honest about your expertise. You're being clear about where your knowledge is deep and where you're learning.

Knowing When You're Being Heard vs. Tokenized

This is important because it's easy to mistake inclusion for actual influence. It's easy to feel gratified that you're at the table without asking whether being at the table actually matters.

I interviewed JJ Singleton for my Advocacy at Work podcast, and he said something that stuck with me. He said if he ever feels tokenized, he brings it up with the organization. He hasn't found an organization yet that hasn't made adjustments based on his feedback. But if they didn't, he said, he'd stop saying yes. He'd tell them why. And he'd move his energy somewhere else.

That's the bar. You should feel heard. Your input should matter. The organization should be responsive when you point out where they're missing the mark. If that's not happening, the problem isn't you. The problem is the organization.

Being at the table but not being heard is actually worse than not being at the table. Because it perpetuates the idea that patient voices are included when they're actually being ignored. It's performative inclusion rather than real partnership.

So as you build your strategic voice and expertise, pay attention to this. Are you being asked for your input and then ignored? Are your suggestions dismissed? Are you only invited when they need a patient story but not when actual decisions are being made? Are you the only patient voice in a room, which can feel isolating rather than inclusive?

If the answer to these questions is yes, it's worth asking whether this is a place where your expertise is actually valued. And it might be worth considering whether your time would be better spent elsewhere. With organizations that actually listen. With organizations that make changes based on patient feedback. With spaces where your voice actually shapes outcomes.

That doesn't mean you should leave the first difficult situation. It means you should go in with eyes open. You should notice when you're being heard and when you're being tokenized. And you should be willing to use your voice to name the difference.

Your Authority Grows

The beautiful thing about transforming personal experience into strategic voice is that it's not a destination. It's a process. It doesn't end when you get your first committee role or your first peer review. It keeps evolving.

Early in my advocacy journey, I was just sharing my story, just being honest about my experience, which felt like the extent of my expertise.

Now I'm reviewing research proposals. I'm advising organizations on patient engagement. I'm mentoring new advocates. I'm helping shape research priorities. I'm testifying before legislators. My voice has authority not just because I'm a patient, but because I've learned how these systems work. Because I've built relationships with people in power. Because I've shown I can think strategically about how patient voices can create change.

But none of that would have happened if I hadn't started where I started. With a $150 gift card. With honest answers to survey questions. With showing up. With saying yes.

So if you're just beginning this journey, don't be discouraged if you feel like you're not yet an expert. You don't need to be. You just need to be honest. You just need to show up. You just need to keep engaging.

Your authority will grow. Not because you'll become a doctor. But because you'll become an expert in your own experience. And you'll learn how to translate that experience into influence. Into voice. Into change.

That's how personal experience becomes strategic voice. Not all at once. But gradually. Through showing up. Through consistency. Through refusing to be tokenized. Through building relationships with people who recognize your value.

And through never forgetting that your story matters. Because it does. Always.

Chapter 6

Research Advocacy
and Peer Review

The $150 That Changed Everything

I got paid $150 for an hour of my time. A company sent me a survey. They wanted my perspective on something. I filled it out. I answered their questions honestly. I shared my experience.

Easy money, I thought.

I didn't realize at the time that I was doing research advocacy. I wasn't sitting on a steering committee. I wasn't reviewing research proposals. I was just answering survey questions and getting paid for my time.

But here's what mattered. I said yes to that opportunity. And then I said yes to the next one. And the next one. These survey opportunities started multiplying. Different organizations wanted to hear from patients. They wanted our perspective. They were willing to compensate us for our time.

That's how it started for me. Not with a grand vision of becoming a research advocate. Not with training or credentials or a strategic plan. Just with being willing to say yes to an opportunity. To being honest about my experience. To understand that my perspective had value in research spaces.

About a year after my diagnosis, around the time I was getting those surveys, I started thinking about more formal research advocacy and applied to be a CDMRP peer reviewer. I missed the deadline that first year. But I applied again the next year and was accepted.

I was invited to be a PCORI Ambassador and attended their annual conference for the first time, where I joined steering committees. Some of these opportunities came from organizations reaching out directly. Many came because I was an ambassador with Fight CRC, and being part of their RATS program—Research Advocacy Training and Support—opened doors to more opportunities.

Years one through three were all about learning. I was a novice. Things came to me and I said yes. Years three and four saw more opportunities, many of them repeated roles with organizations that trusted my work. Year five was when everything seemed to come together. The opportunities solidified. The work deepened. And I started to truly understand what research advocacy actually was.

The Reality of Peer Review

Let me be honest about my first CDMRP peer review experience, because it was overwhelming: so many terms I'd never heard of, the complexities of a government-run program, tight deadlines, prework you have to do, and specific formats you have to use for your responses. It was a lot.

But then I got on the call. The first day was six hours. The second day was another six. After all the formalities and introductions, we started reviewing the first proposal. I was nervous. Really nervous.

And then the other patient reviewer gave her input. And something shifted for me.

Her response was short. She spoke in words I could understand. Not medical jargon. Not research speak. Just her perspective, clearly and simply expressed.

The pressure was off. I realized I didn't need to be an expert in research methodology. I didn't need to understand all the terminology. I just needed to answer as myself. To share my perspective as a patient. To ask the questions a patient would ask.

And here's what surprised me most. The researchers and doctors on the panel were all very appreciative of us being there. They wanted our input. They asked us questions. They treated us as valuable team members.

We finished both days ahead of schedule. The peer review process that was supposed to take all six hours was completed early because the conversations were productive. Because patient perspective actually added value to the discussion.

I'm definitely looking forward to participating again.

What Patient Reviewers Bring

Here's the thing about being a patient reviewer or serving on a steering committee: you're not there to be the expert in research methodology. You're not there because you have an MD or a PhD. You're there because you have something nobody else on that panel has. You have the lived experience of being a patient.

Don't try to be the expert in everything. That's not your role. Use your personal experience and what you've learned from other patients as your source of knowledge.

When researchers are designing a study, they're thinking about scientific rigor. They're thinking about what markers to measure. They're thinking about statistical power and methodology.

What they're not always thinking about is the patient's real-world experience. They might design a study that requires blood draws every week, and from a research perspective, that's fine. However, from a patient perspective, that might mean missing work every week. It might mean a significant burden on someone who's already dealing with treatment.

Patient advocates catch those things. We understand the burden of treatment. We understand what it takes to participate in a trial. We understand what would make a study accessible versus what would make it impossible.

I know that Cologuard was developed based in part on patient input. The issue was clear to patients: a colonoscopy is intrusive. It's time-consuming. It's expensive. The prep is unpleasant. It's not pleasant to talk about. It keeps people from getting screened.

Patients said: there has to be a better way. And researchers listened. They developed a non-invasive test you can do at home. No special prep. No sedation. No time off work. Just a test you can do in the privacy of your own home and mail back to a lab.

That's what happens when patient input shapes research. You get something that's not just scientifically valid. You get something that actually works for patients. That actually gets people screened.

Preparing for Research Advocacy

If you're thinking about getting involved in peer review or steering committees, here's what you need to know.

First, prepare. Read and review all the information they provide before joining. If you don't understand something, ask questions. Don't pretend you know what something means. Ask for clarification.

Second, understand the time commitment and compensation. Know how many hours you're committing to. Know how much you're being paid. And yes, you should be paid. Researchers pay statisticians. They pay consultants. Why shouldn't they pay patients for our expertise?

When I first heard that researchers were compensating statisticians for their time, something clicked for me. If they're paying specialists for their expertise, patients should be compensated for ours. Our time has value. Our expertise has value. Expect to be paid for it.

Third, know that you don't need a medical background. You don't need to understand all the jargon. What you need is the willingness to learn, to ask questions when you don't understand, and to trust that your perspective matters.

Steering Committees vs. Peer Review

There's a difference between peer review and serving on a steering committee, and it's worth understanding.

Peer review is basically reviewing a proposal and giving your input on whether it's good research. Whether it addresses important questions. Whether the design makes sense. Whether the outcomes being measured matter to patients.

A steering committee is different. You're not reviewing a proposal. You're helping shape the research once it's underway. Your role is to help them understand the important factors from a patient perspective. To help them reach as many people as possible. To help them make the trial as successful as possible.

My position on the Natera steering committee is a good example. Natera is developing a diagnostic tool currently in clinical trial stage. My role is to help them think about how it would reach the most people, especially in underserved markets. How it should be marketed to the public. What information should be on the website. What barriers might prevent people from accessing it.

They use our feedback to help shape their go-to-market strategy. How they communicate with patients. What's on their website. What resources they provide.

Will we ever see the exact impact of our feedback? Maybe not. By the time the diagnostic tool completes clinical trials and receives FDA approval, it could be years before we can measure the impact. But I look at it this way: if this tool, even in clinical trial phase, can save one person who wouldn't have been screened by today's methods, it will be worth it for me.

The hope is that it will help millions of people down the road. That's why I do it.

Building Your Research Advocacy CV

Here's something I wish I'd known from the beginning: this IS research advocacy. Take credit for it and start building your research advocacy CV right now.

It's much easier to do this in the moment, as things happen, than trying to put it all together after the fact. Keep track of:

- Surveys you've participated in
- Peer review work you've done
- Steering committee roles
- Advisory panels
- Grant review work
- Conference presentations
- Published papers you've contributed to

Build your CV as you go, because eventually, all of that adds up, becoming evidence of your expertise. It becomes something you can point to when applying for better opportunities.

Finding Research Advocacy Opportunities

So how do you actually get involved in research advocacy? Where do these opportunities come from?

The best way is to get involved with organizations like PCORI or Fight CRC. Show up at conferences. Talk with the pharma companies. Attend webinars. Join professional organizations.

PCORI actively recruits patient advocates. You can apply to serve on their advisory panels. You can volunteer to review research applications. You can attend their workshops and training sessions. Visit their website and look for "Get Involved" or "Volunteer" pages.

Fight CRC's RATS program—Research Advocacy Training and Support— trains advocates and then presents them with ongoing opportunities to participate in research. Being part of that program has been instrumental in my own journey.

Pharmaceutical companies increasingly have patient advisory boards. They want input on everything from clinical trial design to how they market their products. If you have expertise in a particular disease or condition, reach out to companies working in that space.

Professional organizations often have research committees looking for patient input. Medical schools. Research institutions. Cancer centers. They're all looking for patients willing to serve on boards, review studies, or provide feedback on research design.

The National Cancer Institute, the Department of Defense Peer Reviewed Cancer Research Program, ASCO, the FDA—all of these have opportunities for patient involvement in research.

And compensation should be part of the conversation. PCORI expects organizations to budget for compensating patient partners. It's becoming more standard. If an organization isn't offering to compensate you, that's worth asking about or potentially passing on.

Taking Credit and Building Authority

Here's what I want to emphasize because I think it matters: every time you participate in research, every time you contribute your perspective, every time you help shape how research gets designed or implemented, that's research advocacy. That counts. It matters.

Don't downplay it. Don't act like you're "just" a patient. You're a patient expert. Your expertise is valuable. Your perspective shapes research.

The more you say yes to opportunities, the more you show up, the more you contribute, the more your authority grows. Not because you suddenly have credentials, but because you've demonstrated over time that your input has value.

By year five, when people started seeking me out specifically, it wasn't because I'd been to medical school. It was because I'd spent five years saying yes. Showing up. Being consistent. Building relationships. Contributing thoughtfully.

That's how you build research advocacy authority. Not overnight. But over time. Through consistency and genuine engagement with the work.

A Note on What Patient Advocates Can't Do

Let me also be clear about something: there will be things in research spaces that don't make sense to you. Terms you don't understand. Design choices that seem odd. Statistical concepts that feel foreign.

Some of those are things you need to ask about. But some of them are just part of research expertise that you don't have. And that's fine. That's why there are researchers on the panel. Your role isn't to understand everything. Your role is to understand the patient perspective. To ask questions. To push back when something doesn't seem patient-centered.

If they can't explain something in a way that makes sense to you, that might be a legitimate question. Or it might be a limitation of your expertise. You'll learn the difference over time.

The key is being intellectually humble while still trusting your own expertise. You're an expert in patient experience. You're learning as you go in research spaces. Those two things can coexist.

Chapter 7

The Recap and the Transition —From Finding Your Voice to Amplifying Others

How This Book Came to Be

Someone once asked me: "If you could do anything, what would it be?" I didn't hesitate. My advocacy. I wanted to work for an organization engaged with advocacy. I wanted to be in this space full-time.

They suggested I start a podcast. Become a thought leader. Build visibility in the space I wanted to work in.

So I did. I started recording episodes. Built a website. Got things in motion. And then I was offered a job. Life happened. For a few months, the podcast sat there, partially built. But eventually, I made the time, and launched it properly in June 2025. By October 2025, I was regularly publishing episodes.

A few months into the podcast, something became clear. There was so much valuable information flowing through these conversations that people kept telling me I should write a book. Not just once or twice. Over and over. The feedback was consistent: write a book.

And I realized what that book should be about. Not my cancer story. Not just my personal journey. But a guide. A resource. Something that could help thousands of other people who wanted to get involved in advocacy but didn't know where to start or how to navigate it.

This book is that resource.

Learning From Others

I didn't figure all of this out alone. Along the way, I've been fortunate to have mentors and advisors who helped me understand the landscape.

Joe Bullock taught me about opportunities through Savvy, where patients can take short surveys and contribute their perspective. Michael Holtz gave me strategic advice. I remember him telling me something important: if I wanted to stay in government research advocacy, they wouldn't accept me if I worked with pharma companies. That was valuable context as I made decisions about which opportunities to pursue.

I didn't make my choices solely based on Michael's advice, but I kept it in mind. As opportunities came my way, I thought about fit. About what aligned with my goals. About where I could have the most meaningful impact.

That's different from my early years when I said yes to everything. Now I was being more intentional. More strategic. Still saying yes, but saying yes to the right things.

The Mentoring Moment

One of the most rewarding parts of building authority in advocacy is having the opportunity to mentor others. I remember a conversation with a patient advocate who works in research professionally. He was on a research call where he would have done things entirely differently if he'd approached it from the angle of his professional expertise.

I pulled him aside. I said: here's the thing. When you're on these panels as a patient advocate, they want your patient experience. They want your perspective as a patient. Not your professional experience. Those are different hats.

But I also told him: if you feel strongly about something, if you think there's a better way based on both your perspectives, address it with the person running the program. Don't stay silent. But understand which perspective you're bringing to that conversation.

That's the kind of advice I wish I'd had early on. Understanding your role. Knowing what hat you're wearing. Not trying to be everything or know everything, but being clear about what you're bringing to the table.

The Things Nobody Warns You About

If I could go back and give myself advice on day one of this journey, there are three things I'd emphasize.

First: Burnout and Mental Health Matter

You will lose people. You will build relationships with people and then lose them to cancer. It gets harder each time. The more people you come into contact with, the more relationships you build, the more loss you experience.

I've talked about this before, but it bears repeating here. If I want to be angry at cancer for taking Chuck and Lee, I need to be angry at cancer for bringing them into my life in the first place. The relationships were worth it. But the grief is real.

This work is emotionally taxing. You're surrounded by people fighting disease. You're in spaces where the stakes are high. Where people's lives depend on the research being done right. Where you see the gaps in the system over and over.

You need support. Therapy helped me. A decade of mindfulness and meditation practice helped me. Taking breaks from advocacy work is not a failure. It's necessary. It's how to sustain yourself for the long term.

Don't pretend you're fine if you're not. Don't think you have to do this alone. Build your support system. Use it.

Second: Know What You're Passionate About and Let the Rest Go

This one takes time to figure out. There's no shortcut. You learn through trial and error.

When I started, I said yes to everything. Steering committees. Peer reviews. Surveys. Speaking opportunities. Advisory panels. All of it.

Over time, I realized what energized me and what drained me. What felt meaningful and what felt like I was just showing up. Some things excited me. Other things felt obligatory.

You don't have to do everything. You don't have to say yes to every opportunity. But you have to try enough things to know what you actually love doing.

Maybe you'll discover you love mentoring. Maybe you'll love the research side. Maybe you'll love legislative advocacy. Maybe you'll love awareness campaigns. Maybe you'll love community building.

The beautiful thing about advocacy is there are many forms of it. You don't have to be good at all of them. You just have to be passionate about the ones you choose.

Give yourself permission to try things. And give yourself permission to say no to things that don't align with your passion or energy.

Third: Sometimes You Have to Say No

Early in my journey, I talked about saying yes. Say yes to opportunities. Say yes to learning. Say yes to showing up.

That's still true. But here's what I didn't mention. There comes a point where you have to get strategic about your yeses.

You can't do everything. You'll burn out if you try. Your impact will be diluted if you're spread too thin.

So yes, say yes early. Try things. Build your experience. Get your hands dirty. Learn what works.

But as you get more involved, as you build authority, as opportunities multiply, you need to be willing to say no. To choose. To focus.

I have more opportunities available to me now than ever before. And I turn down more than I accept. Not because I don't care. But because I'm committed to doing the work I do accept really well.

Quality over quantity. Impact over volume. Sustainability over burnout.

The Force in Numbers

Here's what I want to emphasize as we move into the next section of this book: advocacy is not a competition.

When I mentor someone new to advocacy. When I help them find their voice. When I guide them toward opportunities that fit them. I'm not losing anything. I'm not being diluted. I'm not weakening my own position.

I'm making advocacy stronger. I'm adding another voice to the chorus. Another perspective. Another person pushing for change.

The force in numbers is real. More advocates means more voices.

More voices means more impact. More impact means real change in healthcare systems, in research priorities, in patient outcomes.

If you're reading this book and you're thinking about getting involved in advocacy, I want you to know something. You're not stealing my seat at the table. The table isn't zero sum. More advocates means we need more seats. It means the movement gets stronger.

That's the mindset we need in advocacy. Not scarcity. Abundance. Not competition. Collaboration. Not gatekeeping. Opening doors.

This is why I'm writing this book. This is why I started the podcast. Not to hoard knowledge. Not to position myself as the expert everyone has to go through. But to democratize access to advocacy. To help people figure out their path faster than I figured out mine.

We need advocates everywhere. We need voices in research. We need advocates in legislative spaces. We need community advocates. We need people doing awareness work. We need fundraisers. We need mentors. We need people building infrastructure.

If this book helps you find your place in that ecosystem, I've done my job.

Wrapping Up Part 2

In Part 2, we've talked about starting your advocacy journey. We've talked about building relationships and managing the weight of loss. We've talked about finding your voice and moving from personal experience to strategic advocacy. We've talked about research advocacy and peer review.

What we've really been talking about is you. Your path. Your voice. Your authority.

Part 3 is different. Part 3 is about the organizations you'll work with. The systems you'll navigate. The landscape you'll operate in.

Because advocacy doesn't happen in a vacuum, but within organizations. Within structures. Within ecosystems.

You now have the foundation. You understand what advocacy is. You understand your why. You understand how to build your voice and your authority.

Now we're going to talk about how to operate effectively within the organizational structures that are already out there. And how to identify which organizations are worth your time and energy.

Because not all opportunities are created equal. Not all organizations are actually committed to patient-centered work. Not all advocacy spaces are healthy.

Learning to navigate that landscape, to choose wisely, and to operate effectively within these systems—that's what Part 3 is about.

Are you ready?

Chapter 8

Choosing the Right Organization: Real Commitment vs. Box-Checking

When you're new to advocacy, opportunities feel like gifts. Someone asks you to join a committee. To participate in a focus group. To serve on an advisory board.

Your instinct is to say yes.

And, early on, I still think you should say yes. Try things. Build experience. But as you get more involved, you need to develop a critical eye. Not all organizations that claim to value patient advocacy actually do.

Some organizations have genuinely embedded patients in their decision-making structures. Their work is shaped by patient input. Their priorities shift based on what patients tell them. Their staff includes people with lived experience. They're willing to advocate even when it's uncomfortable.

Other organizations have patient advisory boards that exist primarily for optics. They check the box. They can say: "We have patient input!" But that patient input doesn't actually influence anything. Decisions are made before patients are consulted. Feedback is thanked and filed away. Nothing changes.

Learning to tell the difference is critical. Because the wrong organization will drain your energy, waste your time, and leave you feeling used.

Power Sharing: Who Actually Has a Voice?

The first thing to evaluate is whether patients actually have power.

This sounds obvious, but it's worth being specific about. Real power means patients sit on boards, steering committees, or leadership councils with real authority. It means feedback from patients leads to visible changes. It means patients aren't just advisors—they're decision-makers.

Box-checking looks like one-off focus groups with no follow-up. It looks like "patient advisory boards" that are symbolic, unpaid, or completely ignored. It looks like patients being consulted after decisions have already been made.

When you're evaluating an organization, ask yourself: Can patients meaningfully influence priorities? Or are they just validating them?

One concrete example: I've been involved with Fight CRC's RATS program—Research Advocates Training and Support. An advocate in the program brought to their attention that it always seemed to be the same people getting the opportunities to attend the major colorectal cancer conferences. The selection process wasn't transparent, and it felt like certain advocates received preferential access.

Instead of dismissing the feedback, Fight CRC listened. They changed the process. They made the submission process more transparent. They ensured that advocates who hadn't had the opportunity to attend previously would get a better chance. That's real power sharing. That's feed-back leading to visible change.

Lived Experience in Leadership

Here's something I notice when I walk into an organization: Who's running things.

Real commitment means leadership includes people with lived patient or caregiver experience. Staff are trained in trauma-informed, patient-centered practices. The organization's advocacy is informed by real patient journeys, not just policy theory or what sounds good in a conference presentation.

Box-checking is when all advocacy is handled by communications or policy teams with no patient background. Patient stories get used for fundraising or PR materials. But the actual strategy? That's decided by people who've never had the experience of being a patient navigating a healthcare system.

When you're evaluating an organization, look at the leadership team. Look at the staff performing the actual advocacy work. Do any of them have lived experience? Not "I know someone who had cancer." But actually, personally, navigated it?

This matters because lived experience changes how you think about problems. A communications person might think the best approach to raising awareness is a social media campaign. A patient advocate knows that awareness without access is useless. A person who's navigated the healthcare system knows the barriers in ways theory can't capture.

Investment: Time, Money, and Staff

You can tell what an organization actually values by how much they invest in it.

Real commitment looks like dedicated budget lines for patient advocacy work. It looks like full-time staff responsible for patient engagement and support. It looks like long-term funding commitments, even when advocacy is inconvenient or controversial.

Box-checking looks like advocacy funded only through restricted grants or during specific awareness months. It looks like one staff member wearing five hats with no real resources to actually do the work. It looks like advocacy disappearing during budget tightening.

Here's the litmus test: Would advocacy survive if it didn't generate immediate ROI or good press?

If the answer is no, you know what you're dealing with. The organization values the optics of patient engagement, not the actual work.

When you're vetting an organization, ask about their budget. Ask whether there's dedicated staff. Ask how long they've been committed to patient engagement and whether that commitment is stable or dependent on external funding.

Willingness to Challenge Systems (Including Their Own)

This is where you see if an organization really believes in patient advocacy or just the idea of it.

Real commitment means the organization speaks out when policies, partners, or systems harm patients. They're willing to risk funding, relationships, or reputation to defend patient needs. They openly acknowledge shortcomings and course-correct.

Box-checking means advocacy is carefully worded to never upset funders, sponsors, or regulators. There's silence on controversial but critical patient issues. There's a defensive posture when patients criticize the organization itself.

I've been fortunate to work with the PAN Foundation, which demonstrates this really well. The PAN Foundation hosts an Advocacy Action Summit where they bring patient advocates together to identify legislative priorities. The organization takes this feedback seriously. After one summit, advocates provided input about the number of legislative asks on Capitol Hill. They felt overwhelmed—asking Congress for too many things at once diluted the message and made it harder to advocate effectively.

Did PAN Foundation dismiss this? Did they defend their original strategy? No. They listened. The following year, they reduced the number of asks based on patient feedback. That's an organization willing to challenge its own approach when patients say: "This isn't working."

When you're evaluating an organization, ask: Do they advocate when it's uncomfortable? Or only when it's safe? Do they defend patients even when it costs them something?

Outcomes Over Optics

One of my biggest pet peeves in advocacy is when organizations focus entirely on activity rather than impact.

Real commitment means tracking outcomes that matter to patients. Quality of life. Access. Equity. Survivorship. It means publishing impact reports that show both successes and failures. It means measuring long-term change, not just activity volume.

Box-checking means metrics are all about the number of campaigns, posts, events, or impressions. Success is defined as "awareness raised" without any evidence of real-world impact. Success is measured internally, not by patient benefit.

Here's the difference. One organization might say: "We reached 50,000 people with our awareness campaign!" Another organization says: "We reached 50,000 people with our awareness campaign, and as a result, screening rates in our target demographic increased by 12%."

The second one is measuring what actually matters.

When you're evaluating an organization, ask them to point to concrete changes in patients' lives. Not activities. Not reach. Not impressions. Actual changes. Better access. Lower out-of-pocket costs. Policy shifts. Improved screening rates. Lives saved.

If they can't answer that question clearly, be wary.

Equity and Inclusion Aren't Afterthoughts

I've seen organizations perform patient engagement in a way that only appeals to the easiest-to-reach patients.

Real commitment means advocacy addresses disparities across race, income, geography, disability, and language. Outreach includes under-represented and marginalized patient populations. Resources are accessible—in language, in cost, in digital access.

Box-checking means DEI language without targeted action. Advocacy centered on the most privileged patient voices. One-size-fits-all patient engagement that doesn't actually reach the people most impacted by health disparities.

Here's the litmus test: Who is missing from the conversation? And does the organization care enough to go find them?

I think about this a lot with advocacy for colorectal cancer, which is the third leading cause of cancer death in the U.S, and early-onset colorectal cancer—in people under 50—is rising. Who gets the advocacy attention? Who gets the research funding? Who gets the aware-ness campaigns?

If the answer is mostly people over 50, mostly white, mostly affluent, then you're seeing selective advocacy. That's box-checking.

Real commitment means asking: "Who isn't in this room? Who isn't being served? What barriers are we creating?" And then actually doing something about it.

Long-Term Relationship Building

One of the things that bothers me most is when organizations use patients as props.

Patients get contacted when a good story is needed. When there's a campaign. When there's a press release to write. Then silence until the next campaign.

Real commitment means maintaining ongoing relationships with patients beyond campaigns. Supporting' patients even when they're not "success stories." Valuing trust over transactional engagement.

Box-checking means patients are contacted only when stories are needed. Engagement drops after events, awareness months, or funding cycles. No follow-up. No feedback loops. No real relationship.

When you're thinking about joining an organization, ask yourself: How will they treat me if I'm not useful to them right now? Will they maintain a relationship, or will I disappear until they need something?

Here's the question that matters: Do patients feel used or supported?

Transparency and Accountability

The last thing you want is to commit your time to an organization and then discover they're not being straight with you.

Real commitment means clear advocacy goals and positions. Transparency about funding sources. Openness about conflicts of interest, especially in healthcare and pharma spaces. Mechanisms for patients to raise concerns safely and know they'll be heard.

Box-checking means vague commitments with no public benchmarks. Defensive or opaque governance. No way for patients to challenge the organization without fear of being shut out.

When you're evaluating an organization, look for clarity. Clear goals. Published positions. Transparent funding. And critically, ask: How would I raise concerns if I disagreed with something? Is there a mechanism for that? Would I feel safe using it?

If the answer is no, that's a red flag.

How to Ask These Questions

So you've identified an organization you're interested in. How do you actually ask these questions without sounding accusatory or suspicious?

During the initial conversation:

"I'm really interested in understanding how patient feedback is actually used. Can you give me a concrete example of a time when patient input changed a decision or a direction?"

This gets at power sharing and outcomes. Their answer will tell you a lot.

About structure and investment:

"Who on your team is responsible for patient engagement? What's their full-time equivalent?"

If someone is performing patient engagement as a side project, that tells you something. If they won't give you a clear answer, that also tells you something.

About their willingness to challenge:

"Tell me about a time you advocated for something controversial. Something that might have cost you."

If they can't think of an example, or if they only talk about safe advocacy, take note.

About outcomes:

"What metrics do you actually track around patient impact? Not reach or awareness—actual outcomes."

Their answer will reveal whether they're measuring what matters. About equity:

"Who participates in your patient engagement? Tell me about the diversity of the group."

If they get defensive or vague, that's a sign they haven't thought deeply about this.

About safety for dissent:

"What happens if a patient disagrees with the organization's direction? How would that be handled?"

Their answer matters. You want to know you can speak up without being punished.

What to Do if You Discover an Organization Is Box-Checking

Sometimes you don't realize until you're already involved. You join a committee, attend a meeting, and only then do you start seeing the patterns.

Feedback gets ignored. Decisions are made without patient input. Your time feels wasted. The organization talks about patient engagement but doesn't actually practice it.

What do you do?

First, give it time. One meeting might not be enough to judge. Some organizations are learning and growing. Maybe this is their first attempt at real patient engagement. Maybe they'll improve.

But if you see a pattern over time, you have a few options. Option 1: Provide direct feedback.

Pull the person running the program aside. Say: "I've noticed this feedback wasn't incorporated. Can you tell me what happened?" Be direct. Be specific. Give them a chance to explain or improve.

Some organizations will respond to this. They might not have realized the problem and will appreciate the feedback.

Option 2: Raise it formally.

Some organizations have mechanisms for patients to raise concerns. Use them. Write it down. Make it official. Some organizations will respond to formal feedback when they wouldn't respond to informal conversation.

Option 3: Step back.

Sometimes the best response is to recognize that an organization isn't a good fit and move on. Your time and energy are valuable. You don't have to give them to an organization that doesn't genuinely value patient input.

There's no shame in this. It's not a failure. It's you being smart about where you invest your advocacy energy.

The Ultimate Question

If I had to sum this all up into one question to ask before committing to an organization, it would be this:

"What have patients changed here because of their involvement?" Not what patients have done. What patients have changed.

Have patients changed the organization's priorities? Changed the way they operate? Changed the direction they were heading? Changed their policies or practices?

If the answer is "nothing"—or worse, if they can't think of an example — you know what you're dealing with. You're dealing with an organization that values the optics of patient engagement, not the real thing.

If the answer is clear, specific, and points to real change, then you might have found the right organization.

Pay attention to that answer. It will tell you everything you need to know.

Chapter 9

Patient-Centered
Strategy in For-Profit
Healthcare Organizations

When I first became involved in research advocacy, I noticed something interesting. The organizations approaching me fell into two different categories.

First, there were nonprofits like Fight CRC and the PAN Foundation. Their mission was broad. They cared about colorectal cancer prevention, early detection, treatment access, affordable healthcare, survivor-ship, funding for research. They were trying to move the needle on all of it.

Second, there were for-profit organizations. Pharmaceutical companies. Diagnostic companies like Exact Sciences. Medical device manufacturers. Their focus was different. They were developing specific products. They wanted patients to know about those products. They wanted feedback on those products from people who actually used them or might use them.

For a long time, I was skeptical of working with for-profits. I worried about conflicts of interest. I worried about being used for marketing purposes. I worried that patient advocacy would be secondary to business interests.

But then I started actually working with them. And I realized some-thing. For-profits can do patient advocacy really well. Not always. But when they do, they do it differently than nonprofits. And understanding those differences matters.

The Fundamental Difference in Focus

Here's the basic distinction. Nonprofits are generally focused on broader issues that impact patients. Fight CRC cares about screening rates, early detection, access to treatment, research funding, survivor-ship support. They're working on systemic change across the entire colorectal cancer ecosystem.

For-profits are generally focused on developing products that help patients, or increasing awareness for their products that help patients. Exact Sciences develops the Cologuard test. They want patients to know about it. They want feedback on it. They want to understand how to make it accessible and useful.

This isn't a judgment. It's just different. And it matters because it changes how you evaluate whether the organization is genuinely committed to patient advocacy.

With a nonprofit, you're asking: "Are patient voices influencing their broader strategy?" With a for-profit, you're asking: "Are patient voices shaping this specific product, and how does it reach people?"

Both questions matter. Both require real patient input. But with for-profits, the focus is narrower.

Understanding the Business Model

Here's something I had to learn: for-profit healthcare organizations exist to make a profit. That's not cynical. That's just the reality. They have shareholders. They have quarterly earnings reports. They have business models that depend on selling products.

This used to bother me. I thought it meant patient welfare would always come second.

But since then, I've changed my thinking. The question isn't whether a for-profit makes a profit. Of course they do. The question is whether making a profit comes at the expense of patient benefit.

Those are two different things.

A company can be profitable and still genuinely committed to patient advocacy. They can make money and still put patient needs first in their decision-making. They can have business objectives and still listen when patients say: "This isn't working for us."

When you're evaluating a for-profit organization, that's the litmus test. Does their profit motive come at the expense of patient benefit? Or can they pursue both?

A for-profit that develops a screening test that catches cancer earlier and is more accessible than existing options is doing something good for patients. The fact that they make money on it doesn't negate the patient benefit.

A for-profit that creates barriers to access so they can maximize profits is prioritizing business over patients. That's a different story.

Understanding this distinction helps you work with for-profits without being naive. You're not pretending they're nonprofits. You're not pretending profit isn't a motivator. You're just asking whether they're willing to balance profit with patient benefit.

Red Flags Specific to For-Profits

There are certain things to watch for when you're working with for-profit organizations. They're red flags that suggest the company might be more interested in using you than genuinely engaging with you.

Red Flag 1: No Compensation

Any for-profit that asks you to participate without paying you or covering your travel expenses should be a major red flag.

Let me be clear: this isn't about greed. This is about respect and value.

If a company is asking for your expertise, asking for your time, asking you to contribute to their product strategy or research, they should be compensating you. They pay their scientists. They pay their researchers. They pay their consultants. Why shouldn't they pay patients for their expertise?

Now, when a for-profit approaches me without mentioning compensation, I ask about it directly: "What's the compensation for this work?" If they hesitate or push back, I know something's off. Either they don't respect the value of patient input, or they're not genuinely committed to patient engagement.

Either way, it's not worth my time.

Red Flag 2: Who Are You Actually Talking To?

When you're invited to participate in a for-profit's patient advisory work, ask yourself: Who am I actually talking to?

Are you talking with marketing and PR teams? Those conversations often feel collaborative, but the goal is to help them sell the product more effectively. That's not necessarily bad, but it's not patient advocacy. It's market research.

Are you talking with researchers, advocacy teams, and doctors on their staff? Those conversations are different. They're trying to understand how their product actually affects patients. They're trying to improve it. They're trying to make sure it's accessible and useful.

The difference matters.

Now, I ask this question directly: "Who will be in the room? What are their roles?" If it's all marketing and communications, I'm cautious. If there are researchers, doctors, and advocacy people involved, that tells me they're taking patient input seriously.

What Good For-Profit Patient Advocacy Looks Like

The best example I can point to is Boehringer Ingelheim.

Boehringer Ingelheim works with Fight CRC's RATS program, but they didn't just create a one-off patient advisory board. They went deeper.

They invited RATS advocates to participate in learning labs. These weren't merely focus groups where we just answered questions, but collaborative sessions where we were actively involved in thinking through their research and approach.

Here's what mattered: they brought their advocacy people to the session. They brought their researchers. They brought their doctors. They created an environment where patient input could actually influence their thinking across different departments.

And then they did something that really stood out. After the session, they asked for our feedback. Not about whether we liked their product. But if the experience was valuable. Whether we felt heard. Whether we had suggestions for how they could do this better.

They were being intentional about patient engagement, treating it as something that required ongoing refinement, not just a checkbox to complete.

And they recognized the work. I've been thanked publicly at conferences for my contributions to their efforts. Not because I need public recognition, but because it signals that they value the advocacy work. They see it as a legitimate contribution, not just a nice thing patients do on the side.

That's what I look for in for-profit organizations. Not perfection. But genuine commitment to making patient input part of how they operate.

The Key Questions to Ask

Before committing to work with a for-profit organization, ask these questions:

1. What's the compensation and will you cover travel?

Don't settle for vague answers. Get clarity on what you'll be paid and whether travel is covered. If they hesitate or push back, that's information.

2. Who am I actually talking to?

Ask for a roster of who will be in the room. Will there be researchers and doctors, or just marketing? Will patient input actually reach the people making decisions, or will it be filtered through a communications team?

3. What specifically are you hoping to learn from patients?

A good for-profit can articulate what they need from patient input. They're not just checking a box. They have specific questions. Specific areas where they want patient perspective. If they can't articulate this clearly, that's a red flag.

4. How will you use the feedback we provide?

This is the critical question. Ask them to point to a previous time when patient feedback led to a change. If they can't think of an example, be wary. This might be the first time they're genuinely listening to patients.

5. Will there be ongoing engagement or is this a one-time thing?

If it's truly about getting patient input, it should be ongoing. Products evolve. Patient needs change. A one-time focus group might be market research. Ongoing engagement suggests genuine commitment.

6. Are there transparency and accountability mechanisms?

In the same way you'd ask a nonprofit, ask a for-profit: If I disagree with something, how do I raise it? Will I be heard? Can I push back without being cut off from future opportunities?

Understanding the Tension

Let me be honest about the tension you'll feel working with for-profits.

You care about patients. You want every colorectal cancer patient to have access to screening. You want people to get diagnosed early. You want treatments to work. You want people to survive.

A for-profit company also cares about these things. But they also care about market share. About profitability. About shareholder returns.

These don't have to be in conflict. A company can develop a product that genuinely helps patients and also make money on it. Cologuard is a good example. It's a screening test that doesn't require a colonoscopy. No prep. No sedation. You can do it at home. That's genuinely helpful for patients. And Exact Sciences makes money on it.

But they can come into conflict. A company might decide to limit a product's access to a certain geographic area to maximize profits there first. Or they might price a product in a way that puts it out of reach for uninsured or underinsured patients. Or they might focus on profitable markets and ignore underserved communities.

Your job as a patient advocate working with a for-profit is to highlight those tensions when they arise. To say: "This pricing strategy leaves out patients who need this most." Or "This distribution plan doesn't reach rural communities where screening rates are lowest."

Sometimes they'll listen. Sometimes they won't. But your job is to make sure patient needs are part of the conversation.

The Value of Diverse Partnerships

Here's what I've learned: you need both nonprofits and for-profits in the healthcare advocacy ecosystem.

Nonprofits can push for systemic change. They can advocate for policy. They can work on screening rates and access. They can say things that might upset funders because they're not dependent on any single company.

For-profits can develop innovative products. They can get those products to market. They can scale what works. When they partner authentically with patients, they can create products that are genuinely useful and accessible.

When both types of organizations are working well, and when they're all listening to patients, real change happens.

The Cologuard test exists because patients said: "Colonoscopy is too much of a barrier." Patient input shaped that product. And now it's available because a for-profit company had the resources to develop it and bring it to market.

That's how the system should work.

A Word About Pharma

I want to specifically address pharmaceutical companies because they deserve special attention.

Pharma companies have a particular history with patient advocacy. They've funded patient organizations to promote their drugs. They've used patient testimonials in marketing. They've been accused of "dis-ease mongering"— creating awareness of conditions so people will buy their treatments.

This history creates legitimate skepticism about pharma patient engagement.

So if you're working with a pharmaceutical company, be extra vigilant about the questions I outlined above. Be especially clear about who you're talking to. Be especially careful about whether your input is actually shaping the product or just being used for marketing.

That said, pharmaceutical companies also develop medications that save lives. They employ researchers who are genuinely committed to improving treatments. They have advocacy teams that care about patients.

The question is whether they're willing to prioritize patient needs over marketing needs. Whether they're willing to listen even when patient feedback won't help them sell more drugs.

When a pharma company says: "We want patient input on how to make treatment more accessible," are they actually asking how to remove barriers? Or are they asking how to convince patients who might other-wise skip treatment to stick with it?

Those are two different things.

Working With For-Profits as Part of Your Strategy

If you decide to work with for-profit organizations, do it strategically.

Don't make them your only advocacy work. Keep a portfolio of advocacy activities. Work with nonprofits. Do legislative advocacy. Do awareness work. Stay connected to the patient community outside of corporate structures.

This keeps you grounded. It keeps you from becoming too invested in any one organization's agenda. It makes it easier to push back when necessary.

Also, build relationships with other patient advocates working with the same company. Share information. Compare notes. If you notice something concerning, you'll have others to talk to who understand the context.

And remember why you're doing this: you're doing it because you believe patient input makes products better. Makes treatments more accessible. Saves lives.

When that's true, you're adding value. When it stops being true, you need to be willing to step away.

The Bottom Line

For-profit healthcare organizations can do patient advocacy well. They can genuinely listen to patients. They can let that input shape their products and strategies. They can create things that help people.

But they can also use patient engagement as a marketing tool. They can ask for input and ignore it. They can compensate poorly or not at all. They can center profit over patient benefit.

Your job is to figure out which category they fall into. To ask hard questions. To set clear expectations. To walk away if those expectations aren't met.

When you do that well, you can partner with for-profits in ways that genuinely serve patients. And that's worth doing.

Because at the end of the day, if a product helps patients, and a for-profit company is willing to listen to patient input to make that product better and more accessible, that's a partnership worth having.

The profit motive doesn't negate the patient benefit. It just means you have to be more vigilant about making sure patient needs stay central to the conversation.

And that's something you're equipped to do.

Chapter 10

Creating Authentic
Patient Advisory Boards

If you work in any healthcare organization, you've probably heard the phrase "patient advisory board." It sounds good. It sounds like the organization is listening to patients. It sounds progressive and patient-centered.

But I've been on patient advisory boards where I spent two hours in a meeting and nothing I said mattered. I've been on boards where the organization brought us in to validate decisions they'd already made. I've been on boards where diversity existed on paper but not in practice.

I've also been on boards where my input actually shaped decisions. Where leadership listened. Where being a patient advocate meant something beyond showing up and sharing your story. The difference between those two experiences comes down to how the organization set up and runs the board.

If you're leading an organization and thinking about creating a patient advisory board, or if you're trying to improve one that already exists, this chapter is for you. That's because there's a right way to do this, and there are a lot of wrong ways that still look good on the surface.

Start With Purpose, Not Optics

Here's where most organizations go wrong from the start.

They decide they need a patient advisory board because it looks good. Because it's trendy. Because competitors have one. Because they want to demonstrate they're patient-centered.

And then they go recruit some patients and expect magic to happen. It doesn't work that way.

Before you recruit a single person, you need to be able to answer three questions in writing:

- What decisions will this board influence?
- What authority does it have?
- What will change because this board exists?

If you can't answer those questions clearly, stop. Don't recruit yet. Figure this out first.

Because if those answers are fuzzy, your recruitment will default to finding "nice storytellers" instead of true advisors. You'll end up with people who are good at sharing their narrative but not necessarily good at thinking strategically about systemic change. And then you'll be surprised when they want more influence than you planned to give them.

Be clear about scope from the start. If the board is advisory only, say that. If it has voting power on certain decisions, say that. If it can influence budget or strategy, be explicit about it.

Clarity about authority prevents a lot of misunderstanding down the road.

How to Actually Recruit Patient Advisors

The best channels for recruiting patient advisors are those where trust already exists.

Start with existing patient networks. Support groups. Peer mentors. Patient navigators. These are people already engaged in the community. They have credibility with other patients. They're used to having difficult conversations.

Partner with clinicians and social workers who know patients beyond the ones who are "good communicators." Sometimes the most valuable advisors are quiet. They don't perform well in meetings. But they have deep wisdom about what patients actually need.

And work with community-based organizations serving underrepresented populations. If you want diverse voices on your board, you can't just make an open call and hope marginalized patients show up. You have to build relationships with organizations already trusted by those communities and co-recruit together.

What you should avoid is equally important.

Don't hand-pick only patients who already agree with leadership. That's not an advisory board. That's a fan club.

Don't recruit exclusively from donors, ambassadors, or brand advocates. These people have already decided they like your organization. You need people willing to push back.

And don't recruit based on "who's available." Recruit based on "who's needed." If your board needs someone with experience navigating insurance barriers, go find that person. Don't just invite whoever can make the meeting.

What Qualities Actually Matter

Not every advisor needs every quality. But your board as a whole should reflect all of them.

Lived experience plus reflection: The person can articulate not just what happened to them, but why it mattered. They understand their experience isn't universal. They can translate their individual story into systemic insight. This is different from just being a good storyteller.

Systems awareness: They can distinguish between individual failure and systemic failure. They ask "Who else is impacted?" not just "What happened to me?" They understand their particular problem might point to a larger issue that affects many patients.

Constructive honesty: They'll speak up even when it's uncomfortable. They can critique without burning the room down. They can disagree without being disagreeable. This is crucial because you need people willing to say hard things.

Collaborative mindset: They're open to other patient perspectives. They can disagree without invalidating others. They understand that different patients have different needs and that's okay.

Reliability: They show up. They follow through. They respect time and process. This might sound basic, but it matters. You need advisors who are committed to the work.

Here's something important: don't select for "polish." Some of the most valuable advisors don't sound like spokespeople. They might be quieter. They might not have the perfect words. But they see things others miss.

If you're only recruiting people who present well, you're excluding a lot of wisdom.

Building Actual Diversity

Diversity doesn't happen accidentally. It requires intentional design.

First, compensate your advisors. Seriously. If you don't pay them, you've already excluded anyone who can't afford to work for free. You've excluded single parents. You've excluded people living paycheck to paycheck. You've excluded a lot of the people most impacted by health inequities.

Offer multiple participation formats. Virtual, asynchronous, translated. Some people can't make meetings in person. Some people work irregular hours. Some people speak languages other than English. If you want diverse participation, you have to remove barriers.

Partner with trusted community organizations to co-recruit. Don't just post an open call. Build relationships with organizations already trusted by communities you're trying to reach.

And explicitly name which perspectives are missing. Don't just hope they show up. Say: "We need people with experience navigating rural healthcare systems. We need uninsured or underinsured patients. We need young adults just diagnosed. We need family caregivers." Then recruit for those specific needs.

What doesn't work: having one "diverse" seat on the board. That's tokenism. That person becomes the voice for an entire community, which is unfair and ineffective.

Also, don't expect marginalized patients to self-nominate into spaces that might not be safe. You have to actively recruit them. You have to build trust. You have to demonstrate that their voices will be valued.

Here's the key mindset shift: equity in patient advisory boards isn't just representation. It's access plus safety. You need both.

Structure That Works

Based on what I've seen work well, here's the structure I'd recommend:

Size: 10 to 15 advisors. Large enough for diversity of thought, small enough for real conversation.

Meeting frequency: Quarterly or bi-monthly, depending on your goals. If you're making major decisions, meet more often. If it's more advisory and strategic, quarterly works.

Mix: Include both patients and caregivers. Include a variety of ages, health conditions (if not disease specific), urban and rural perspectives, different ethnicities. Think about lived experience with healthcare access, socioeconomic status, disability status. Build a board that actually reflects the patients you serve.

Term limits: Generally, two years is a good timeline. But build in options for people to continue beyond two years if they wish, and if it's working. The key is to ensure that at least one-third of the board comprises new members, which keeps perspectives and ideas fresh. If your entire board rotates every two years, you lose institutional knowledge. If nobody rotates, you get groupthink.

Meeting format: Most meetings should be virtual. But there are reasons to gather in person, especially if you're meeting with board members or senior leadership. Sometimes in-person builds relationships in ways virtual meetings don't.

Integration Into Decision-Making

Here's where a lot of boards fail: the patients give input, but leadership does whatever it planned anyway. And nobody ever tells the patients what happened to their recommendations.

Fix this with a decision log.

Publish what you heard from the board. What you changed because of their input. What you didn't change and why. Make this public and visible. Let the board see their impact.

Also, be clear about the reporting structure. The advisory board should report to someone with real authority, usually an advocacy manager or researcher, and that person should report to the president or division head for that product or program. If your patient advisory board reports to the communications department, patients will correctly sense they're not influencing anything real.

Don't expect advisors to know everything about your organization. They're not employees. But for what they're involved with, give them regular updates. Keep them informed about progress. Show them the connection between their input and outcomes.

The goal is to make patient advisors genuine partners in shaping your work. Not employees. Not volunteers. Partners.

What Not to Do

There are several mistakes I see organizations make over and over.

No real authority: Patients give input and leadership ignores it. There's no feedback loop. Patients never hear what happened to their recommendations. Fix this with transparency. Publish a decision log. Show what changed.

Emotional extraction: Organizations repeatedly ask patients to share trauma with no support, no boundaries, no follow-up. Then they use those stories externally without meaningful benefit to the patient. This is exploitation, not engagement. Fix this by moving from storytelling to problem-solving. Trauma is not a requirement for participation.

Over-professionalizing patients: Teaching patients to "sound more strategic." Filtering out emotion and dissent. Turning advisors into unpaid staff. Stop this. Let patients be patients. Strategy is your job.

Truth is theirs. You need their honest perspective, not a sanitized version.

Homogenization over time: The board slowly fills with the same type of voice. New or dissenting perspectives stop showing up. Groupthink sets in. Fix this with term limits, staggered rotations, and intentional refresh cycles. Bring in new voices on purpose.

No internal readiness: This is the hardest one to fix because it's cultural. Your staff aren't trained to hear criticism. Leadership is defensive. Patient input is seen as "nice to have" rather than essential. Here's the hard truth: if your organization's culture can't tolerate critique, don't start a patient advisory board yet. You'll just frustrate everyone.

Real Examples

I've been on boards that got it right. And boards that missed the mark. Let me share what I've learned from both.

Board that got it right (Pattern 1):

Patients had voting power on program priorities. Advisors were paid and supported. Leadership regularly said: "We changed this because the board told us to." When patients disagreed publicly, leadership backed them.

Why it worked: Patients weren't advisors in name only. They were co-owners of outcomes. That changed everything about how people participated.

Board that got it right (Pattern 2):

Patients were involved before study design. Plain-language materials were non-negotiable. One patient vetoed a protocol that would have increased burden without real benefit. And leadership listened.

Why it worked: Patient impact outweighed academic convenience. That's the hierarchy that needs to exist.

Board that missed the mark (Pattern 1):

High-profile patient stories. No influence on actual policy or budget. Advisors rotated out once they became too critical.

Failure mode: Advocacy used as brand insulation, not accountability. Board that missed the mark (Pattern 2):

Diverse on paper, unsafe in practice. Marginalized advisors repeatedly ignored or talked over. Leadership cited "consensus" that didn't actually exist.

Failure mode: Representation without power is exploitation.

The Gut Check

Here's how to know if your patient advisory board is real or performative.

If your organization says: "Our patient advisory board helps us validate our work," they're probably doing it wrong.

If they say: "Our patient advisory board regularly forces us to rethink our work," they're much closer to getting it right.

The difference is whether the board is there to confirm what you already believe, or to challenge and make you better.

You need the second one. Patients need the second one. Healthcare needs the second one.

For Patient Advisors Reading This

If you're on a patient advisory board and aren't sure whether you're having real impact, look for these signs:

- Do you get regular updates on what happened to your recommendations? Can you see the connection between what you suggested and what changed?
- Are you asked for your perspective before decisions are made, or after?
- Do you feel safe disagreeing with leadership?
- Are you compensated fairly for your time?
- Is your board diverse, or is it a pretty homogeneous group?
- Are you asked to repeatedly share trauma, or are you asked to solve problems?

If you're saying no to most of these, you might be on a board that's more about optics than impact. You can either try to address it directly with leadership, or you might decide your time is better spent elsewhere.

Your expertise is valuable. Make sure you're using it somewhere it actually matters.

The Bottom Line

Creating an authentic patient advisory board takes real intention. It requires clarity about purpose. It requires commitment to equity. It requires leadership willing to be influenced by patient voices.

It's not easy. But it's essential.

Because when you get it right, patient advisory boards are one of the most powerful tools healthcare organizations have. They make you smarter. They make you more responsive. They make you better at serving the communities you exist to serve.

And that's what it's all about.

Chapter 11

Community Management as Advocacy Infrastructure

I've spent 17 years building communities. Before I ever called myself a healthcare advocate, I was helping people connect with each other around shared interests and purposes. I was building spaces where people felt welcome. Where they could be heard. Where their voice mattered.

It took me a while to realize that community management and advocacy are deeply connected. In fact, community management is the infrastructure that makes real advocacy possible.

When you strip away the jargon, community management in an advocacy context is simple: it's people coming together around a shared purpose to work towards a shared outcome and impact.

That's it. But getting that right changes everything about how advocacy actually works.

What Community Management Actually Means

Many organizations use the word "community" loosely. They have a Facebook group. They send out newsletters. They host webinars. And they think that's building community.

It's not. That's broadcasting. That's distribution. That's one-way messaging.

Real community is something different. It's relational. It's reciprocal. It requires the organization to genuinely listen and respond. It requires advocates to feel like their voice shapes what happens next.

In my 17 years of community management, I've learned that the best communities share certain characteristics. They're welcoming. They're supportive. They provide impact with purpose. They're consistent. They listen with empathy. They share authentic stories.

When an organization gets those things right, community becomes the backbone of their advocacy work. It's where relationships form. It's where advocates find each other. It's where real change gets built.

When an organization gets those things wrong, community becomes a liability. It becomes a place where people feel used. Where their voice disappears into a void. Where they lose faith in the organization.

The difference between those two outcomes depends on how seriously the organization takes community management.

The Six Principles of Strong Advocacy Communities

Welcoming

This sounds basic, but it's critical. Newcomers need to feel welcome. They need to know this is a space for them, even if they're newly diagnosed, newly engaged, newly angry about the healthcare system.

Welcoming means removing barriers to entry. It means explaining how things work. It means having people who actively greet newcomers and help them understand the community's norms and values.

It also means being intentional about who you're welcoming. Are you creating a space that feels safe for people of color? For LGBTQ+ patients? For people with disabilities? For people living in rural areas? For people who don't speak English as a first language?

Welcoming communities do this intentionally. They don't just hope marginalized patients show up. They actively work to make those patients feel like they belong.

Supportive

Community isn't just about advocacy. It's about people supporting each other through shared experiences.

In the best patient communities, someone newly diagnosed can ask a question and get ten responses from people who've walked that path. People share resources. People share their fears. People celebrate wins together.

This support is what keeps people engaged over the long term. It's what makes the difference between a patient feeling isolated and a patient feeling like they're part of something bigger than themselves.

Organizations that build truly supportive communities understand that sometimes people need help before they're ready to advocate. Some-times they need to process their diagnosis. Sometimes they need to know they're not alone. And that's okay. That's part of the community's purpose.

Impact With Purpose

Here's where community bridges to advocacy. Real communities aren't just about venting and support. They're about doing something with that shared experience.

A supportive community helps you feel less alone. An impact-focused community helps turn your experience into change.

Man Up to Cancer provides support for men navigating cancer so they don't have to isolate. But they also create opportunities for those men to advocate together. To speak at conferences. To influence research. To mentor other men.

That's impact with purpose. The community isn't an end in itself. It's a foundation for making things better.

Consistent

People need to know what to expect. They need to know that if they show up, something real will be there. That conversations will happen. That responses will come. That the organization will follow through.

Consistency builds trust. It tells people their time and energy are valued.

This means regular meetings or gatherings. It means responding to messages within a reasonable timeframe. It means being reliable about what you say you'll do. It means showing up even when it's not convenient.

Communities that lose momentum often do so because they lose consistency. The organization gets busy. Meetings get canceled. Messages go unanswered. And people stop showing up because they learn not to expect anything.

Listening With Empathy

This is where a lot of organizations fail. They create a space for people to participate, but they don't actually listen.

Listening with empathy means hearing not just the words someone is saying, but understanding the experience behind those words. It means recognizing that different people have different needs and perspectives, and that's valuable.

It means asking questions to understand better. It means responding thoughtfully, not defensively. It means being willing to change course based on what you hear.

Real listening also means being transparent about what you've heard. Reflecting back what you understood. Explaining how that feedback influenced decisions. Closing the loop so people know their voice mattered.

Authentic Stories

The best communities run on authentic stories. Not polished testimonials. Not carefully curated narratives. But real people sharing real experiences.

This authenticity is what creates connection. It's what makes people feel seen and understood. It's what builds trust.

Organizations that rely on perfect stories or only highlight "success stories" miss something important. People need to hear from people at different points in their journey. People who are angry. People who are still figuring things out. People who are struggling.

When communities share authentic stories, people realize their own story matters. That they have something to contribute, even if they're not "inspirational," polished or further along in their journey.

Building the Listening Infrastructure

Principles are important, but they mean nothing without actual systems and structures to support them.

If you're building an advocacy community, you need to create intentional listening infrastructure. This looks different depending on your context, but the goal is the same: to make sure the community's voice is heard and acted upon.

Create Spaces for Connection

This could be an online forum where patients can ask questions and support each other. It could be monthly virtual meetings where advocates gather to discuss challenges and opportunities. It could be annual in-person conferences where the community comes together.

The format matters less than the consistency. People need to know where to find each other and when.

The best communities have multiple formats because different people engage in different ways. Some people are comfortable in large group settings. Others need smaller conversations. Some people prefer asynchronous written communication. Others want real-time dialogue.

If you only offer one format, you're automatically excluding people.

Provide Training, Resources, and Opportunities

A listening community doesn't just listen. It equips people to act.

This might mean providing training on how to participate in research. How to advocate to policymakers. How to tell your story compellingly. How to navigate healthcare systems.

It means sharing resources. Research summaries. Policy updates. Information about clinical trials.

It means creating opportunities for people to get involved. To serve on committees. To speak at conferences. To mentor others. To contribute their expertise in meaningful ways.

When people feel equipped and have clear pathways to involvement, they engage more deeply. They feel agency. They become advocates rather than just community members.

Gather Timely Feedback

Ask your community what's working and what's not. Do this regularly, not just when something goes wrong.

This could be through surveys. Through one-on-one conversations. Through open forums where people can share ideas. Through feedback sessions after events.

The key is timeliness. Ask for feedback while something is fresh. Respond quickly to what you hear. Let people see that their input led to changes.

Provide Status Updates and Progress Reports

Close the loop. Tell people what you've heard, what you're doing about it, and when you'll have updates.

If someone suggests the community needs a rural patient perspective, tell them you heard that. Tell them you're reaching out to rural-focused organizations. Tell them you'll update them in three months about what you've learned.

This transparency is crucial. It shows people that feedback isn't disappearing into a void. It shows that their voice is being taken seriously.

Bring Feedback Into Decision-Making

This is the critical step that a lot of organizations miss. They gather feedback, but then they don't actually use it.

If your community says they need more mental health resources, actually find those resources or connect people with them. If they say they feel unheard in certain contexts, work on changing those contexts. If they say the current meeting format doesn't work for them, change the format.

Sometimes you won't be able to do what people ask. That's okay. But explain why. Explain what you're doing instead. Explain when you might be able to revisit it.

The goal is to show that feedback matters. That people's voices shape what happens next.

Real Examples of Community Done Right

COLONTOWN and Man Up to Cancer are both excellent examples of communities that get this right.

COLONTOWN

COLONTOWN is an online support community for colorectal cancer patients and caregivers. Their tagline is "where hope meets science," and that captures what they do.

They have clearly defined rules about what's acceptable in the community. They hold to those rules consistently. And they're deeply responsive to member feedback. That doesn't mean they do everything people ask. But they explain their decisions with empathy and understanding of the differences in people's needs.

What makes COLONTOWN work is that they understand their purpose. They're not trying to be everything to everyone. They're creating a safe space for CRC patients to get support, share information, and connect with others who understand their journey.

Because of that clarity, they can make decisions that serve their community well. And because they listen and respond to feedback, members feel valued and heard.

Man Up to Cancer

Man Up to Cancer is a community for men navigating cancer as patients or caregivers. They do amazing work creating spaces where men don't have to isolate through their cancer journey.

But they also do more than support. They create opportunities for the men in their community to engage in advocacy. To speak. To influence research. To mentor other men.

What makes them work is that they genuinely understand their members. They know that men might not show up if it feels like a support group. They create community through activities, retreats, and connections. And then, within those communities, advocacy naturally emerges.

They're consistent. They're welcoming. They share authentic stories. They provide impact opportunities. And they listen to their community and evolve based on what they hear.

What NOT to Do

There are patterns I see organizations repeat that destroy community.

Using Community as a Marketing Tool

This is the biggest one. When organizations treat community as just another marketing channel, people feel it.

One-way messaging. Information that people can already get from your website or social media. Calls to action that primarily benefit the organization rather than the community.

This isn't community. This is transactional. And people know the difference.

Real community requires reciprocity. The organization gives and takes.

It listens as much as it broadcasts. It benefits the people in the community, not just the organization.

Inconsistency

Communities fall apart when organizations lose consistency. Meetings get canceled. Messages go unanswered. Regular content updates stop. The energy drops.

If you're going to build a community, commit to showing up consistently. That's the bare minimum.

Ignoring Difficult Feedback

Some organizations build community until people start saying things they don't want to hear. Then they get defensive. They dismiss the feedback. They silence the person who raised it.

This kills community faster than almost anything else.

If you can't handle being criticized by the people you serve, you're not ready for community. Build that internal capacity first.

Only Centering Certain Voices

Some communities inadvertently create hierarchies. Certain people are elevated. Certain voices are amplified. Others are marginalized.

This happens when you only share "success stories." When you only invite the most eloquent advocates to speak. When you don't actively work to include people at different stages of their journey.

Real community includes everyone. The newly diagnosed. The angry. The grieving. The hopeful. The uncertain.

Community as the Foundation of Advocacy

Here's what I've learned over 17 years of building communities: when you get community right, advocacy becomes sustainable.

People stay engaged longer. They're more likely to take action. They're more willing to speak up and push for change. They have each other's backs.

When you get community wrong, advocacy becomes transactional. People feel used. They burn out. They leave. And the organization loses both the people and the wisdom they carried.

Community is where advocates find their voice. Where they realize their experience isn't unique. Where they understand that what happened to them points to something bigger that needs to change.

Community is also where organizations learn what actually matters to patients. What the real barriers are. What needs to change.

When community is working, it's a feedback loop. Advocates share their experiences and perspectives. Organizations listen and respond. That response shapes what advocates push for next. Those impacts create new stories that get shared in the community.

It's virtuous. It's powerful. And it's the foundation of real change.

Building Community With Intention

If you're leading an organization and thinking about how to build community, start with purpose.

Why are you bringing people together? What do you hope will happen? How will you know it's working?

Then build the infrastructure to support that purpose. Create spaces for connection. Provide training and resources. Listen with empathy. Close loops. Show that feedback matters.

Be consistent. Be welcoming. Be authentic. Be willing to be influenced by the people in your community.

Do that, and you'll build something powerful. Something that sustains advocacy for the long term. Something that actually changes things.

Because at the end of the day, advocacy isn't something a single person does. It's something a community does together.

And that's where the real power lies.

Chapter 12

Content, Communications, and Storytelling

I've been creating content about advocacy for years now. Through a podcast. Through writing. Through speaking. Through social media.

And I've learned something important: how you communicate about advocacy matters just as much as what you're trying to communicate.

Bad advocacy content can undermine your message. It can make people tune out. It can make your advocacy feel inauthentic or self-serving.

Good advocacy content can move people. It can inspire action. It can create change.

The difference comes down to understanding who you're talking to, what you're trying to accomplish, and how to tell your story in a way that actually lands.

What Makes Advocacy Content Good

Good advocacy content varies depending on what type of advocacy you're engaged with. Research advocacy looks different from legislative advocacy. Awareness campaigns look different from fundraising appeals.

But there are principles that hold across all of it.

Talk to the patient directly, not to patients as a group

This sounds subtle, but it changes everything about how you write and speak.

When you talk to "patients" (plural, abstract), your language becomes different. It becomes more formal. More distant. More about policy and systems.

When you talk to a patient (singular, specific), your language becomes more direct. More personal. More about their individual experience and what they can actually do.

I notice this with a lot of advocacy content. Organizations write about "the patient experience" or "patient needs" in ways that feel abstract and clinical. They're not talking to patients. They're talking about them.

Good advocacy content talks to the person reading or listening. It addresses them directly. It assumes they care enough to pay attention. It respects their intelligence.

Focus on what change you can make, not what they can do for you

This is crucial. The worst advocacy content is transactional. It's asking something of people without giving them something first.

"We need your donation." "We need your story." "We need you to call your representative."

Those asks might be necessary. But they can't be the main point of your content.

Good advocacy content starts by offering something. Offering perspective. Offering hope. Offering a pathway forward. Offering information that helps someone make a better decision about their health.

Then, if there's an ask, it comes naturally. It's an extension of what you've already offered, not a bait-and-switch.

Use plain, easy-to-understand language

Some research still has complex medical terminology. That's okay. But explain it. Translate it into words people actually use.

A lot of advocacy content falls into the trap of using legal and professional language. It sounds official. It sounds credible. But it also sounds distant and inaccessible.

Good advocacy content is written the way real people talk. It uses everyday language. It explains concepts simply. It doesn't assume expertise on the part of the reader.

This doesn't mean dumbing things down. It means respecting that your audience is intelligent but might not have medical training. You're a translator. You're helping them understand something complex in a way that actually makes sense.

Good Storytelling in Advocacy

Many people think good storytelling in advocacy means telling the best version of your story. The most inspiring. The most triumphant. The most shareable version.

That's wrong.

Good storytelling in advocacy means sharing your entire story. Not the highlight reel. The real thing.

It means not framing your experience the way social media wants. The best side. The rosy outlook. The sanitized, feel-good version.

It means being honest about the hard parts. The scary parts. The uncertain parts. The angry parts.

Here's how I approach it: I start by understanding what point I'm trying to get across. What action do I want people to take? What under-standing do I want them to have?

Then I look at my story and ask: Which part of my experience actually demonstrates that point? Which part brings that home in a way that data or policy language can't?

Then I tell that part of my story. Fully. Honestly. Without filtering it into something more palatable.

Using data and vulnerability together

When I'm advocating in front of legislators, I often start with data. Here are the facts. Here's what the research shows. Here's what's broken about the current system.

Then I follow with a relatable part of my story. This is what that data means in a human life. This is what it felt like to navigate this broken system.

Then I explain why this matters. Not just to me, but to others. Why this is a problem that needs solving. Why it matters right now.

And then, if there's an ask, I make it clear. Here's what needs to change. Here's what I'm asking you to do about it.

That combination is powerful. Data gives you credibility with policy-makers. A relatable story gives them something to remember and some-thing that sticks. Explaining the broader why helps them understand the stakes. And a clear ask tells them what action you want them to take.

If you're being vulnerable—really vulnerable, sharing real struggles and real fears—you build credibility in a different way. But here's the key: you have to be consistent about it.

I believe in this so much that I have a tattoo on my arm that says: "Let the world feel your heartbeat." But that doesn't mean oversharing everything or performing vulnerability for social media.

What it means is showing up authentically. I could sit behind my computer, make up stories, and share them consistently. People might believe me. For a while.

But that's not what I do. I show bits and pieces of my actual journey along the way. Through my podcast. Through my social media. Through conversations. Over time, people see the consistency between the story I tell and the person I actually am.

That's where real credibility comes from. Not from perfection. Not from always saying the right thing. But from showing up authentically, repeatedly, over time.

Different Formats Serve Different Purposes

I create content in multiple formats: podcasts, Substack blog, social media, speaking engagements. And I've learned that each format has different strengths.

Social Media

Most people won't read a long-form post on Instagram or other social platforms. They'll scroll past it. They'll engage with something shorter, snappier, more visual.

I use social media for short updates. Photos from advocacy events. Quick insights. Moments from my personal life and advocacy journey mixed together.

Social media is where I share bits and pieces of what I'm working on. It's not where I do deep-dive education about advocacy. It's where I direct people to other places I perform that work.

Substack/Email/Blog

Substack is my home base for written advocacy content. This is where I publish longer pieces. Where I can go deeper into a topic. Where I share content that wouldn't fit on social media.

People will read long-form content on Substack or via email if they've chosen to be there. They've opted in. They expect substance. They have time to read it.

This is where I can share complicated ideas. Where I can tell a story with nuance and detail. Where I can explain something complex in a way that requires more than a few sentences.

Podcast

The podcast lets people listen to 30 minutes of conversation while they're doing other things. Driving. Working out. Doing dishes.

That's time they probably wouldn't spend reading a 30-minute article. But they can listen to a podcast episode.

The podcast format also creates intimacy. There's something about hearing someone's voice, hearing the real conversation, that builds connection in a way written content doesn't.

My podcast lives on my Substack and is also distributed to podcast platforms. People who come to the podcast know what they're getting: advocacy-focused conversations with people doing real work in this space.

The Ecosystem

These formats work together. My social media directs people to my Substack. My podcast episodes are shared on social media, which directs people to listen on the podcast platform or read the blog. My written content gets referenced in my speaking engagements.

It's an ecosystem. Each format serves a different purpose, but they all point toward the same mission.

Knowing Your Audience

My audience is anyone interested in advocacy. It could be a newly diagnosed patient who's wondering how to get involved, or an organization trying to figure out how to improve patient engagement.

But I tailor my content based on who I'm talking to.

When I share content for an organization, I use titles and questions that are relevant if you're an organization. What makes an authentic patient advisory board? How do you integrate patient feedback into decision-making? How do you compensate advisors fairly?

When I share content for patients, I use titles and questions that are relevant if you're a patient. How do you find advocacy opportunities? How do you build your voice? How do you know if an organization is genuinely committed to your input?

The content is different because the needs are different. Understanding your audience means understanding what they're trying to figure out. Then you address that directly.

What Actually Resonates

I'm still early in my podcast journey. But I'm noticing something. The episodes that seem to resonate most are the ones where I let my guests talk. Where they share things they haven't shared in other places.

It's not about me asking the perfect questions or providing the perfect commentary. It's about creating space for someone to say something real. Something that matters to them. Something that might change how people think about advocacy.

When that happens, people respond. They share the episode. They tell me it meant something to them.

It's a reminder that good content isn't about being perfect. It's about being real. It's about letting people see themselves in what you're sharing. It's about creating space for genuine conversation.

Always Include a Call to Action

Good advocacy content should have a call to action. Even if the action is small.

If I'm sharing about colorectal cancer screening, I'm reminding people to get screened. If I'm talking about research advocacy, I'm pointing people toward opportunities to get involved. If I'm sharing someone's story, I'm asking people to do something with what they've learned.

The call to action should flow naturally from the content. It shouldn't feel tacked on. It should feel like the next logical step based on what you've just shared.

Sometimes the call to action is immediate. "Call your representative today." Sometimes it's longer-term. "Start thinking about how you might want to get involved in advocacy." Sometimes it's reflective. "Consider what your advocacy might look like."

But there should always be something. Because content without action is just information. And there's already plenty of information out there. What's scarce is information that moves people to do something different.

Authenticity Is Non-Negotiable

I've noticed something about advocacy content that doesn't land. It often feels like it's trying too hard. Trying to be inspiring. Trying to be professional. Trying to be perfect.

The best advocacy content I've encountered is the opposite. It feels like someone just being real. Sharing what's actually true for them. Not performing. Not filtering. Not trying to be something they're not.

This is harder than it sounds. Especially when you're creating content in professional spaces. There's pressure to sound a certain way. To present yourself a certain way. To emphasize certain parts of your story and minimize others.

But that pressure is what makes advocacy content feel inauthentic. And inauthentic content doesn't move people.

So commit to authenticity. Even when it's uncomfortable. Even when you're not sure what people will think. Even when it would be easier to sand down the rough edges and present a smoother version of yourself.

The rough edges are where the real connection happens.

Creating Content With Purpose

Before you create any piece of advocacy content, ask yourself:

- What do I want people to understand after they engage with this?
- What action do I want them to take, if any?
- Who specifically am I talking to?
- Why does this matter? Why now?

Answer those questions clearly, and the rest of the content becomes clearer. You know what to include. You know what to leave out. You know what story to tell.

Create content that answers real questions people have. Content that moves people toward understanding or action. Content that respects your audience's time and intelligence.

Do that, and you're creating advocacy content that actually matters.

Because advocacy content isn't just about broadcasting your message. It's about creating space for people to see themselves in your work. To understand why it matters. To realize what they might do about it.

That's the power of good content. And that's worth getting right.

Chapter 13
Measuring and Communicating Impact

One of my favorite moments in advocacy work happens every year at the PAN Foundation's Advocacy Action Summit.

The advocates gather and PAN Foundation shares the numbers from the previous year's advocacy work. How many letters and calls were made to Congress. How many included personal stories. How many states and districts were covered.

We hear these numbers as we're getting ready to spend a day on Capitol Hill, meeting with legislators and their staff. Making calls. Sharing stories. Pushing for policy change.

There's this palpable sense of accomplishment in the room. You can feel it. Advocates realize the scope of what they accomplished last year. They understand that their individual call or letter was part of something much bigger.

And that understanding inspires them. They go into their Hill meetings energized and motivated. They go home inspired to send more emails, make more calls, and visit their representatives' home offices. They return next year ready to do even more.

That's what good impact reporting does. It takes individual effort and shows how it connects to collective change. It celebrates what was accomplished. And it motivates continued engagement.

But a lot of organizations miss this opportunity. They measure the wrong things. Or they measure the right things but don't communicate them in ways that matter to advocates.

What NOT to Measure: Vanity Metrics

Before we talk about what to measure, let's be clear about what doesn't matter.

How many members you have. How many posts you've published. How many likes or replies those posts received.

These are vanity metrics. They look impressive in a report. They make the organization feel productive. But they don't tell you anything about whether your advocacy actually created change.

An organization could have 100,000 social media followers and zero legislative impact. Could have published 500 posts and never influenced a single research priority. Could have received thousands of likes and not saved a single life.

Vanity metrics measure activity. They measure reach. But they don't measure impact.

Real impact measurement is harder. It requires thinking about what actually matters in your specific context. It requires being willing to report numbers that might be smaller but more meaningful.

What TO Measure: Real Impact Metrics

Real metrics depend on what type of advocacy you're doing.

For Awareness Advocacy

What matters is reach and impressions. How many people got the message? Not how many liked it, but how many actually received it?

This matters because awareness is the goal. You're trying to get information in front of people. If your goal is to raise awareness about colorectal cancer screening, you need to know how many people your campaign reached.

But even here, there's a caveat. Reach is a means to an end. The real question is: Did that awareness lead to action? Did people get screened? Did people talk to their doctors? Did awareness translate into behavior change?

When you can measure that—when you can show that your awareness campaign led to increased screening rates—that's real impact.

For Research Advocacy

What matters is how many advocates participated. Not in a vague sense, but specifically. How many patient advisors sat on steering committees? How many participated in peer review? How many helped shape research design?

But again, the real question is deeper. Did that patient input change the research? Did it lead to different outcomes being measured? Did it make the study more accessible to patients? Did patient involvement improve the research in concrete ways?

For Legislative Advocacy

What matters is how many meetings took place. How many calls and emails were made. How many states or districts were covered.

But the real impact question is: Did anything change? Did a bill move forward? Did a policy shift? Did funding increase?

You can make a thousand calls and nothing changes. You can make fifty calls and shift a legislator's vote. The number of calls matters less than the outcome they produced.

For Fundraising Advocacy

What matters is how much was raised and how many people donated.

But the real impact question is: What did that money do? Did it fund research that led to breakthroughs? Did it provide resources to patients who couldn't afford treatment? Did it increase access or improve outcomes?

I remember working with No Kid Hungry and they had a powerful approach to this. They didn't just say "We raised $100,000." They said "$1 connects a child with 10 meals." It wasn't about the dollars raised. It was about how many mouths could we feed. How many children would have access to nutrition because of that funding.

That's the difference. Money raised is a metric. Money actually helping people is impact.

How I Measure My Own Impact

I measure my own advocacy impact by outcomes that actually matter to me.

How many of my friends get screened for colorectal cancer? That's a real metric. That's my personal contribution to preventing cancer deaths. I keep track of this. I know the number.

Is it a perfect metric? No. I know more about screening outcomes than most advocates because people tell me. But there are probably people I influenced who never told me they got screened. So my actual number is probably several times higher than what I officially track.

But I also know I can't account for everything. I spent 2.5 years in treatment. During that time, my main focus was surviving. It wasn't keeping detailed records of every person I influenced to get screened. Life happens. Measurement isn't always perfect.

I keep a CV of my advocacy projects. Every committee I've served on. Every research panel I've participated in. Every conference I've spoken at. Every publication I've contributed to.

I keep track of proclamations I receive. How many cities turn blue each March for colorectal cancer awareness because of campaigns I've been part of.

These metrics matter to me because they're connected to my goals. I want to prevent colorectal cancer deaths. I want to influence research. I want to increase awareness and screening. These metrics track whether I'm actually accomplishing those things.

The Challenge: Attribution and Long Timeframes

Here's what makes advocacy impact hard to measure: attribution is complicated. Impact often takes years. And the work is often collective.

The screening age for colorectal cancer was lowered from 50 to 45. That's a massive public health win. It means more people will be screened earlier. More cancers will be caught at earlier stages. More lives will be saved.

But how do you measure the advocacy impact of that change? Which organizations should take credit? Fight CRC did legislative advocacy. COLONTOWN provided community support and shared patient perspectives. Research institutions conducted the studies that supported the recommendation. Clinicians advocated for the change within their professional organizations.

That change took ten years. And the work of many organizations working together.

In year one of advocacy, how does an organization report impact? "We're working toward a change that might happen in a decade." That doesn't look impressive in an annual report.

This is why so many organizations fall back to vanity metrics. They're easier to track. They're easier to report. They look impressive even if they don't mean much.

But here's the thing: advocates deserve to know the real impact they're having, even if it's complicated. Even if it takes years. Even if attribution is messy.

Communicating Impact: Make It Real

The best impact reporting I've seen comes from organizations that understand advocates want to know their work matters.

The PAN Foundation shares detailed numbers about legislative advocacy. How many letters and calls. How many personal stories were included. This matters because it helps advocates see the scope of their collective impact.

Both PAN Foundation and Fight CRC publish annual reports specifically for their advocates. Not glossy donor reports full of sanitized stories. Reports that show advocates what actually improved because of their work.

On one of my steering committees, they do something simple but powerful. At the beginning of each meeting, they share some of the feedback from the last meeting that was actually used. They don't get into fine details. But they say: "Based on your feedback, we were able to do this."

That simple acknowledgment tells you that you were heard. That your input is helping create impact. That you're not just showing up to meetings where nothing changes.

That's how you communicate impact in a way that motivates advocates. Not just statistics. But the connection between advocate input and actual change.

What Makes Good Impact Reporting

Good impact reporting has a few characteristics.

It's honest: It doesn't overstate impact or hide failures. If something didn't work, it says so.

It's specific: It points to concrete changes, not vague improvements. "We improved access" is less powerful than "We reduced out-of-pocket costs by 30% for uninsured patients."

It acknowledges collective impact: It recognizes that advocacy is rarely the work of one person or one organization. It gives credit generously.

It connects to mission: The metrics reported are connected to what the organization actually cares about, not just what's easy to measure.

It celebrates advocates: It shows advocates the specific impact their participation created. It makes them feel like part of something bigger.

It's transparent about timeframes: It's honest about what takes years. It doesn't just report quick wins. It gives context about long-game advocacy.

It motivates future action: Good impact reporting doesn't just look backward. It looks forward and shows what's possible if advocates stay engaged.

The Patient Perspective: How You Know You Matter

If you're an advocate serving on a board or committee, here's how you know if your voice actually matters.

- You get regular updates on what happened to your recommendations. Not vague updates. Specific information about what changed because of what you said.

- You see feedback loops. You suggest something. The organization investigates. They come back and tell you what they found. They implement changes or explain why they can't.

- You feel heard in the room. People take your comments seriously. They ask follow-up questions. They don't dismiss your perspective.

- You see your input reflected in actual decisions and changes, not just acknowledged politely.

- You're compensated fairly for your time and expertise.

If most of these are true, you're in an organization that's measuring impact—even if they don't call it that. They're tracking whether patient input leads to change. And that's the metric that matters.

Moving Beyond Metrics to Meaning

Here's what I want to emphasize: advocacy impact measurement isn't really about the numbers.

It's about knowing that your work matters. It's about seeing the connection between what you did and what changed. It's about under-standing that you're part of something bigger than yourself.

When PAN Foundation advocates see how many calls were made to Congress, they're not just seeing a number. They're seeing proof that their individual effort was part of a collective movement. They're feeling the power of many people working together toward the same goal.

When I know that more than 50 of my friends got screened because of my advocacy, I'm not just tracking a statistic. I'm recognizing that I've probably prevented cancer deaths. I've changed lives.

That's what impact measurement is really about. It's about making the invisible visible. It's about showing advocates that their work matters.

So measure what matters. Report it honestly. Celebrate it. And watch what happens when advocates understand the real impact of their engagement.

Because that's when advocacy becomes sustainable. That's when people stay engaged for the long haul. That's when real change happens.

Chapter 14

The Business Case for Advocacy

There's a misconception that talking about the "business case" for advocacy somehow dilutes the mission. That it's cynical or self-serving to acknowledge that patient advocacy also benefits organizations.

It's not. In fact, the opposite is true.

When organizations understand that genuine patient advocacy strengthens their mission, their operations, and their sustainability, they're more likely to invest in it seriously. When they see advocacy not as a feel-good add-on but as essential to who they are and what they accomplish, they do it better.

The business case for advocacy isn't about putting profit over patients. It's about recognizing that advocacy done well serves both. It strengthens the organization while creating real change for the communities they serve.

The Nonprofit Advantage: PAN Foundation

I've had the privilege of working with organizations that truly under-stand this. The PAN Foundation is a perfect example.

PAN started in 2004 as a financial assistance organization. They help patients afford medications. Over nearly 20 years, PAN has helped 1.3 million people, providing more than 4.5 billion dollars in financial assistance across 80+ different programs.

That's vital work. But when Amy Niles joined as Director of Alliance Development in 2014, she asked an uncomfortable question: Why aren't we doing more?

The organization had something most nonprofits don't. They had direct relationships with hundreds of thousands of patients who had lived experience of access barriers. They understood the systems breaking down. They knew what needed to change.

So PAN decided to move beyond financial assistance into policy advocacy. They would channel the voices of the patients they served into systemic change.

It wasn't an easy sell. Some board members resisted. "Waste of time. Waste of resources. You're not going to change anything. Why bother?" they said.

But Amy persisted. And what happened next illustrates exactly why the business case for advocacy matters.

The Long Game: Ten Years to Medicare Reform

PAN spent roughly a decade advocating for Medicare Part D reforms. The barrier was clear and brutal. Before 2022, Medicare beneficiaries faced no cap on out-of-pocket drug costs. Patients were spending

$5,000, $10,000, $15,000 or more annually on medications.

It was catastrophic, exactly the kind of systemic barrier PAN's mission demanded they address.

But nothing changed. Year after year, PAN advocated. They shared stories from affected patients. They educated policymakers about the human impact. They built relationships with Congressional offices. And nothing happened.

The work felt thankless. But PAN kept showing up.

Then, in August 2022, the Inflation Reduction Act passed. And it included key Medicare reforms that capped out-of-pocket costs for the first time.

That victory didn't happen because of PAN alone. It was a collective effort by patient advocates, nonprofits, policymakers, and grassroots activism. But PAN's sustained advocacy—bringing patients' voices to Congress, educating lawmakers, building relationships over a decade—was part of what made it possible.

Here's why this matters from a business perspective. PAN could have given up. Could have decided that policy advocacy was too difficult, too slow, too uncertain to justify the resources. They could have stuck solely to financial assistance.

But they didn't. Why? Because advocacy strengthened their organization's mission. Because advocacy gave their funding bodies concrete evidence that PAN was addressing root causes, not just treating symptoms. Because advocates became ambassadors for PAN, expanding their reach and deepening their impact.

The business case worked. Advocacy made PAN stronger, more relevant, more mission-driven.

How Organizations Grow Through Advocacy

There are concrete ways that authentic patient advocacy strengthens organizational sustainability.

It builds community loyalty: Patients who engage in advocacy become invested in the organization's mission. They're not just receiving services. They're partners in change. That creates the kind of loyalty that transactional relationships never could.

When PAN created their Advocacy Action Summit, it started with 40 advocates. The following year, 65. The year I participated, 85. This year it will grow again. Why? Because advocates come back. Because they feel like they're part of something bigger. Because the organization listened to them and their feedback influenced what happened next.

It expands reach and impact: Patient advocates have networks. They have communities. They have credibility within their own circles that no organization could buy.

When Exact Sciences partnered with Fight CRC to create the State Grant Program, they didn't just fund local events. They enabled Fight CRC to replicate national-level advocacy work across multiple states. That expanded reach benefited both the organization and the for-profit company. It also genuinely served more patients.

It improves program design: When organizations listen to patient voices, they build better programs. They understand barriers they wouldn't have seen from the inside. They learn what actually matters to the communities they serve.

This isn't just nice. It's strategically smart. Organizations that listen to patients make better decisions. They waste less money on programs that don't work. They invest more in programs that do.

It strengthens fundraising and partnership opportunities: Funders increasingly want to support organizations that demonstrate genuine patient engagement. Partners want to work with organizations that walk the talk.

When you can show that patient voices shaped your strategy, improved your programs, and drove your impact, funders notice. Partners want to align with you.

The For-Profit Angle: Exact Sciences

For-profit organizations face a different business case calculation. Their primary obligation is to shareholders, not patients. But authentic patient advocacy can actually strengthen their business model.

Exact Sciences provides a good example. They developed Cologuard, a non-invasive at-home screening test for colorectal cancer. It's a genuinely innovative product that removes barriers to screening. You don't need a colonoscopy. You don't need sedation. You don't need to take time off work. You do it at home.

But developing that product required understanding about what patients actually needed. That required listening to patient advocates.

When Bryan Goettel first came to Exact Sciences, the company didn't even have a dedicated advocacy department. It was all under public relations. But as evidence emerged about rising colorectal cancer cases in people under 50, there was a clear need for a different approach.

Exact Sciences invested in building authentic relationships with patient advocates. Not to use them for marketing. But to genuinely understand the problem they were trying to solve.

That investment strengthened their product. It informed their go-to-market strategy. It helped them understand real barriers to screening that no amount of marketing research alone could have revealed.

And here's the business case part: when patients trust an organization, they use their products. When patients advocate for an organization's mission, they become ambassadors. When organizations have genuine credibility with the communities they serve, they outperform competitors.

The investment in authentic advocacy wasn't altruistic. It was strategically smart. It made their business stronger.

The Key Distinction: Mission-Alignment vs. Transactional Relationships

The business case for advocacy only works when it's authentic. When the organization is genuinely committed to patient benefit, not just using patients for brand building.

This is where for-profit organizations face a unique challenge. How do you work with patients without it feeling like exploitation?

According to Bryan Goettel, the answer is trust-building. "We have to work to build that level of trust for people to see that we're in this for more than just trying to get more people to utilize our products."

How do you build that trust? Through sustained commitment. Through partnership, not extraction. Through recognizing that patient advocates are partners, not props.

At Exact Sciences, they've demonstrated this through the Cologuard Classic golf tournament, which has evolved into a platform bringing together 17 different colorectal cancer advocacy organizations and 360+ survivors and loved ones. They've demonstrated it through the State Grant Program with Fight CRC, a sustained, seven-year partner-ship that funds state-level advocacy work.

These aren't one-off initiatives. They're sustained commitments. They show that Exact Sciences is in this for the long term, not just the next quarter's earnings report.

Contrast that with organizations that use patient stories in marketing, extract patient testimonials for campaigns, and then disappear when the campaign ends. That's transactional. That's not genuine partnership. And it doesn't build the trust that creates real business value.

What Doesn't Work: Misaligned Incentives

There are organizations that understand the business case but get it wrong. They invest in advocacy, but in ways that don't align with patient benefit.

Maybe they fund only the research that reflects well on their company, not the research that answers the hardest questions. Maybe they support advocacy organizations, but only if those organizations never criticize them. Maybe they create patient advisory boards, but don't actually listen to them.

These approaches might generate short-term goodwill. They might look good in marketing materials. But they don't build the deep trust that creates real value.

And they're fragile. The moment patients realize they're being used, the moment they see their input isn't actually influencing anything, the trust evaporates. The advocacy becomes a liability instead of an asset.

The organizations that win are the ones that truly align their business incentives with patient benefit. The ones willing to listen even when it's uncomfortable. The ones willing to invest in advocacy knowing it might take ten years to see results.

The Role of Mission Clarity

Both PAN Foundation and Exact Sciences succeed because they have clear missions and stay true to them.

PAN's mission is making sure everyone can afford and access the care they need. Their advocacy work is rooted in that mission. Everything they do—financial assistance, advocacy, education—serves that mission.

At Exact Sciences, the mission is removing barriers to colorectal cancer screening. Their product serves that mission. Their advocacy work serves that mission. They invest in patient advocates not because it's good PR, but because it helps them understand and address barriers.

Mission clarity is what prevents organizations from getting confused about incentives. It's what keeps advocacy grounded in patient benefit rather than drifting into extraction.

If you're leading an organization and considering investing in patient advocacy, start here. What is your mission? What are you actually trying to accomplish? How does patient advocacy serve that mission?

If you can't answer those questions clearly, you're not ready for advocacy yet. And your patients will know it.

The Sustainability Question

Here's the hard truth about nonprofit advocacy: it requires sustained commitment and resources.

Amy Niles had to educate the PAN Foundation board about why advocacy mattered. She had to fight for resources when board members wanted to question the value. She had to keep showing up even when legislative efforts failed year after year.

That's the cost of authentic advocacy. It's not fast. It's not guaranteed. It requires an organization willing to invest in work that might take years to show results.

But here's the flip side: organizations that commit to genuine patient advocacy become more resilient. They build deeper communities. They attract mission-driven supporters. They create impact that justifies their existence.

The business case isn't that advocacy is cheap. It's that advocacy, done well, creates value that far exceeds the cost.

Saying No

I have one more insight Amy shared that matters for the business case. Organizations have to be willing to say no.

Funders might want PAN to focus on specific issues or measure impact in specific ways. Donors might have preferences that don't align with PAN's mission. But PAN's leadership needs to maintain clarity about their mission and values.

"You can't just take money and not have the transparency for both the funder and yourself as an organization to be like: 'Hey, we're not aligned,'" Amy explains.

This kind of integrity—staying true to mission even when it means declining resources—is what allows advocacy organizations to maintain the trust of both their donors and patient advocates. It's harder in the short term. But it pays dividends in the long term because it signals that you're serious about your mission. That patient benefit isn't negotiable.

The Bottom Line

The business case for advocacy is simple. Organizations that listen to patients, partner with them authentically, and let that input shape their work become stronger.

They become more effective. They become more resilient. They become more trusted. They create deeper impact.

This isn't about cynically using patients to strengthen the bottom line. It's about recognizing that when you serve patients well, when you listen to them, when you partner with them to create change, everyone wins.

Patient voices are heard and they see real impact. The organizations strengthen their mission and sustainability. The systems change.

That's the real business case. And it's worth every investment an organization makes in doing it well.

Chapter 15

Burnout, Boundaries, and Self-Care in Advocacy

I haven't experienced full burnout yet. But I've had instances where I've needed to step back. Where the work that usually fuels me started feeling heavy. Where I realized I needed to pause before I could move forward again.

Those moments taught me something important. Burnout doesn't announce itself with a dramatic collapse. It creeps in quietly. And if you're paying attention, you can catch it before it takes you down.

This chapter is about recognizing those signs. Setting the boundaries that prevent burnout. And taking care of yourself so you can sustain advocacy work for the long term.

Because advocacy is a marathon, not a sprint. And marathons require pacing.

The Unique Grief of Healthcare Advocacy

There's something about this space that's unlike any other. It's not just about people leaving organizations or moving on to other work.

People die.

In advocacy spaces, you build relationships with people. You get to know them. You work alongside them. You care about them. And then cancer takes them. Or their disease progresses. Or complications arise. And they're gone.

This loss is relentless. It's not a one-time thing. It's a pattern. The longer you're in advocacy, the more people you know, the more loss you experience.

I had to learn how to hold that. How to grieve without it consuming me. How to keep showing up when the work brings you into constant contact with death.

It took me about a year to really process this. I remember thinking: "If I want to be angry at cancer for taking them, I need to be angry at cancer for bringing them into my life in the first place."

Because here's the truth. The relationships were worth it. Even though they ended in loss. Even though grief is the price of those connections. They were worth it.

But that doesn't mean grief doesn't hurt. It does. And you have to find a way to carry it without letting it paralyze you.

Understanding Your Energy

Not all advocacy work affects you the same way. Some work energizes you. Some work drains you.

I've learned to pay attention to the difference.

Some conversations fuel me. They remind me why I do this. They connect me to purpose. Those conversations, I can have over and over. They don't deplete me.

Other conversations drain me. They're important conversations. They matter. But they exact a cost that demands time to recover from.

I've known advocates who need to process a lot. Who need to talk through their fears, grief, and anger. That's valid. That's necessary. But it's not always my role to be the person they talk to.

Here's what I've learned: if someone needs more support than I can authentically give them, maybe there's a different person who would be better for them. Maybe there's a therapist, or a support group, or a different advocate who has capacity in that moment.

This isn't about abandoning people. It's about honest assessment. Can I show up for this person in the way they need? If yes, I do. If no, I help them find someone who can.

All advocacy takes some of your energy. But some takes more than others. I try to stick with work that doesn't feel like it's draining me. Work that feels like it's fueling me. That's where I'm most effective anyway.

The Privilege Paradox

Something shifted for me when I reached no evidence of disease. For 2.5 years, I was in active treatment. Cancer was my primary focus. My advocacy work fit around that.

Then I got the news I'd been hoping for. No evidence of disease. I was no longer in treatment.

And I felt guilty.

Who was I to share with other patients if I wasn't actively fighting cancer anymore? What right did I have to offer hope or guidance or support when I was no longer in the trenches?

That guilt almost stopped me from continuing my advocacy work.

I saw a therapist for about nine months to work through this. And something shifted during that time. People started telling me how much my continued advocacy meant to them. How inspiring it was. How it gave them hope.

I realized I was coming from a place of privilege. My treatment had worked. I was granted the outcome many people pray for. And by withdrawing, by staying silent, I wasn't providing hope or knowledge or guidance to people who still needed it.

The opposite was true. My story—the story of someone who got NED, who continued to advocate, who proved that advocacy doesn't end when treatment does—that story had power.

It took therapy to help me see that. It took hearing from other people how my presence mattered. And it took a shift in perspective. I wasn't taking space away from people in active treatment. I was offering a different kind of hope. A different perspective.

But I wouldn't have reached that point without professional help. Without someone trained to help me work through the guilt and the grief and the identity shift.

Warning Signs of Burnout

If you're involved with advocacy work, watch for these signs. They're indicators that you might be heading toward burnout.

Tiredness: Not the kind you recover from with a good night's sleep. But a persistent fatigue. A sense that even when you rest, you're not fully restored.

Lack of motivation: The work that used to excite you feels like an obligation. You're showing up, but you're not present. You're going through the motions.

Irritability: You're more easily agitated than usual. Small things bother you. You snap at people who don't deserve it. Your patience is shorter.

Uncertainty: You start questioning whether your work matters. Whether you're making a difference. Whether it's worth the cost.

Note: This is different from the uncertainty that comes with trying something new. When you take on a new type of advocacy, uncertainty is normal. But if you're feeling uncertain about work you've been doing for a while, that might be a warning sign.

When you notice these signs, that's when you need to step back. Not forever, necessarily. But enough to give yourself space to recover.

Sometimes that's temporary. Sometimes you step back and return refreshed and ready to continue.

And sometimes you step back and realize you're not coming back. That this work isn't serving you anymore. That you need to move on to some-thing else. That's okay too. You don't owe advocacy work your life. You don't owe organizations your participation if it's no longer right for you. Stepping back can become stepping away, and that's a legitimate choice.

Self-Care Practices That Actually Work

I've learned that self-care isn't about spa days and bubble baths. Those are nice, but they're not what sustains advocacy work over the long term.

Real self-care is about practices that help you process what you're experiencing. That help you stay grounded. That help you maintain perspective.

Mindfulness and meditation: I've been practicing mindfulness for about a decade. It's not about clearing your mind or achieving perfect peace. It's about noticing what's happening without judging it. About creating some space between stimulus and response.

When you're in advocacy work, especially in spaces dealing with grief and loss, that space is crucial. It gives you room to feel what you're feeling without being consumed by it.

Community with others who understand: In Man Up to Cancer, I have other advocates I can reach out to. People who have walked similar paths. People who understand the unique challenges of this work.

They've taught me so much about how to handle burnout, survivors' guilt, grief. And they've done it by simply sharing their own experiences. The same way they supported me when I was in treatment.

That reciprocal support—where you're both giving and receiving—is different from extracting support from someone. It's sustainable. It's real.

Professional help: Sometimes you need more than community can provide. You need someone trained to help you process trauma, grief, and identity shifts.

I spent nine months with a therapist working through guilt and shame around my own survival. That was necessary work. It helped me move forward in ways I couldn't have done alone.

If you find yourself struggling, seeing a therapist isn't a sign of weak-ness. It's a sign of wisdom. It's taking care of yourself so you can continue showing up for others.

Knowing what fuels you: Pay attention to which types of advocacy work feel energizing versus draining. Which conversations leave you depleted versus inspired.

Then organize your work accordingly. Not perfectly—sometimes you have to do work that drains you because it matters. But whenever possible, spend your energy on work that fuels you.

Boundaries: The Most Important Self-Care Practice

The most important thing you can do to prevent burnout is set boundaries. And then actually keep them.

Saying no: You can't do everything. There will be more opportunities than you have capacity for. You have to get comfortable saying no to things that don't serve you or that would overextend you.

This is hard. It feels like you're leaving work undone. But saying yes to everything is a faster path to burnout than saying no to some things.

Time boundaries: Decide when you're available for advocacy work and when you're not. Maybe that's not checking emails after 6 PM. Maybe that's designating certain days as advocacy-free. Maybe that's taking breaks between projects.

Your brain and body need rest. Not just sleep, but actual time away from the work. Without it, you'll burn out.

Emotional boundaries: You can care deeply about people and their struggles without taking on their emotional burden. You can support someone without being their primary source of support. You can be present without absorbing all of their pain.

Taking breaks: Sometimes the most important thing you can do for your advocacy is to step away from it for a while. A week. A month. A season.

This isn't giving up. It's refueling. It's giving your emotional reserves time to replenish. It's giving yourself space to remember why you started this work in the first place.

And here's what I want to be clear about: if you step back and later realize you don't want to come back, that's okay too. You don't owe the work your life. You don't owe organizations your continued participation. If advocacy work is no longer serving you, if it's taking more than it's giving, you have permission to leave. Completely. There's no shame in that. There's no failure in that. Sometimes stepping back becomes stepping away, and that's a legitimate choice.

What Organizations Should Know

If you're leading an organization and have patient advocates working with you, there is a responsibility to recognize and address burnout.

Watch for the warning signs: tiredness, loss of motivation, irritability, uncertainty about the work.

When you notice these signs in an advocate, address it. But do it privately and with care. Don't call them out in a meeting. Don't make them feel like they're failing.

Instead, reach out. Ask how they're doing. Ask if they need a break. Ask what support they need.

Some advocates will need to step back temporarily. Honor that. Hold their spot. Welcome them back when they're ready. Don't make them feel guilty for needing rest.

Some advocates might need to shift what they're doing. Maybe they've been engaged with legislative advocacy and it's drained them. Maybe they'd energize more through community work. Listen to what would work better for them.

And some advocates might need to step away entirely, at least for a while. That's okay too. The work will still be there when they're ready to return.

The organizations that care well for their advocates are those that sustain impact over the long term. The ones that burn through advocates are those that don't prioritize this work.

Sustaining Advocacy

Here's what I want to emphasize: advocacy is a marathon. You can't sprint the whole way.

You have to pace yourself. You have to take care of yourself. You have to set boundaries that allow you to keep showing up, year after year.

The loss is real. The grief is real. The emotional toll is real. And it's worth it. But only if you're taking care of yourself while you do it.

Watch for the warning signs. Set the boundaries. Seek the support. Take the breaks. Practice the self-care that actually sustains you.

Because we need advocates who are in it for the long haul. We need people who show up consistently. People who have the capacity to keep fighting. People who take care of themselves so they can take care of others.

That's not selfish. That's essential.

And that's what this chapter is really about. It's about recognizing that taking care of yourself is part of the advocacy work. It's not separate from it. It's central to it.

You can't pour from an empty cup. So fill your cup. Protect it. Rest it. Refuel it.

And then keep showing up. For as long as you can. In whatever form that takes.

Because the world needs your advocacy. But only if you're taking care of yourself while you do it.

Chapter 16

Navigating Conflicts and Difficult Conversations

Conflict is inevitable in advocacy work. You're bringing together people with different experiences, different priori-ties, different perspectives. You're working within systems that don't always prioritize patient benefit. You're asking for change from organizations that might not want to change.

Conflict happens. The question is how you handle it.

Over the years, I've learned that most conflicts aren't as complicated as they seem. And many conflicts can be avoided altogether if you know what to watch for.

The Self-Promoters: Spotting Fakes

There are people who call themselves advocates but aren't really advocating. They're promoting themselves. Or selling something. A diet. A membership. A course. A supplement.

These people use advocacy language. They talk about patient empowerment, community, and change. But underneath, they're running a business. They're building a brand around a disease or condition so they can sell something.

Over the course of my 17 years in community work and five years in healthcare advocacy, I've learned to spot these people pretty quickly.

How? Pay attention to what they're actually asking for. Are they asking for systemic change that benefits all patients? Or are they asking for change that benefits their product or their business?

Are they sharing science-based information? In today's world, you can find just about any "evidence" that will support your position. Most of it is anecdotal and not scientific. Real evidence comes from rigorous research. From peer-reviewed studies. From data that's been tested and validated. If someone is promoting solutions based only on anecdotal evidence or cherry-picked information, that's a red flag.

Are they transparent about their conflicts of interest? Or do they hide them?

Once you identify these people, the answer is simple: don't associate with them. Don't promote them. Don't share platforms with them. Don't lend your credibility to their work.

This isn't mean. This isn't exclusionary. This is protecting the integrity of advocacy work. This is making sure that patient voices aren't being exploited for someone's personal gain.

Most of the time, I just quietly distance myself from these people. No confrontation. No drama. Just a decision not to collaborate or amplify their work.

Keeping Politics Out of Patient Advocacy

One of the fortunate things about my advocacy work is that most of the organizations I work with keep politics out of the conversation. Or they do a very good job of not sharing political leanings and keeping the focus on the issues we're all asking for.

But I have encountered advocates who let their personal political beliefs get in the way of the work.

When that happens, I remind them why we're here. We're here because patients deserve access to screening. Because research should be patient-centered. Because healthcare should be affordable. Because people shouldn't die of preventable cancers.

Those issues transcend politics. They matter regardless of who you voted for or what party you belong to.

I've heard over and over from legislative aides who work on the Hill that when you politicize your message, it isn't heard. If it is, it's not taken seriously. It's the worst thing you can do in a meeting with policymakers.

Think about it from their perspective. A legislative aide is managing dozens of issues. They're trying to figure out which ones matter to their boss and their constituents. When you walk in with a message that's wrapped in partisan politics, you've automatically limited who will listen. You've made your issue tribal. You've turned something that could unite people across party lines into something divisive.

When you make advocacy political, you lose allies. You alienate people who might otherwise support your cause. You turn something that could unite us into something that divides us.

If someone pushes back and wants to keep bringing up their personal political beliefs, I let them know they're free to express those opinions. But good legislative advocacy doesn't focus on who you voted for or what party you belong to. It focuses on what you're asking for. It focuses on the issue.

The strongest advocacy work I've seen keeps politics secondary to the mission. It says: "Regardless of your politics, we can agree on this." And then it focuses on that agreement.

Healthcare shouldn't be a partisan issue. Preventing cancer shouldn't be a partisan issue. Helping patients afford medications shouldn't be a partisan issue. When you keep the focus on the issue—not the politics—you create space for real change.

Having Difficult Conversations With Organizations

I haven't experienced what I'd call a conflict with organizations. But I have had difficult conversations. Conversations where I told an organization something they might not have wanted to hear.

The first time I did this, I remember being nervous. Would they get defensive? Would they shut me out? Would there be consequences?

I told Fight CRC that I thought they had invested in a community plat-form but were wasting their money in the way they were using it. I had feedback about how they could be using it more effectively.

I told PAN Foundation that I thought they had too many legislative asks when I attended my first Advocacy Action Summit. I thought we should focus our efforts more strategically.

Here's what surprised me: neither of these conversations was confrontational. And that's because I wasn't approaching them confrontationally. I was coming from a place of trying to be helpful.

I wasn't saying: "You're doing this wrong." I was saying: "Here's what I'm observing. Here's what I think could work better. I'm sharing this because I want to see your work be as effective as possible."

When you frame feedback in such a way, people are more likely to hear it. They're more likely to take it seriously. They're more likely to act on it.

How to Find the Right Person

One practical thing that helped me: I didn't always know who to approach with my feedback. So I asked.

With Fight CRC, I didn't know who handled the community platform. So I talked to people I did know and asked them to connect me with the right person. They did. And then I had a productive conversation.

This approach does two things. First, it ensures your feedback reaches someone who can actually act on it. Second, it shows respect for the organization. You're not going around behind people's backs. You're not complaining in public. You're seeking out the right channel and having the conversation there.

That approach has worked well for me.

When Advocates Disagree

I haven't seen major conflicts between advocates, but I've heard about them secondhand. Sometimes advocates just don't get along. Some-times they have different approaches or different priorities. Sometimes past hurts create tension.

When that happens, from what I've observed, they just don't work together. They operate in separate spaces. They don't collaborate on certain projects. But they don't make it a public drama. They maintain professionalism. They respect the work the other person is doing, even if they're not doing it together.

That seems like a healthy approach. Not every advocate needs to work with every other advocate. Not every organization needs to partner with every other organization. Sometimes the healthiest thing is to acknowledge that you're not a good fit and move on.

I'm not comfortable sharing secondhand stories about specific conflicts because I didn't witness them myself. But the pattern I've observed is: when advocates or organizations have tension, the ones who handle it well are those who address it privately, directly, and with honesty. The ones who make it public or try to drag others into it tend to create more problems than they solve.

The Most Important Question: Is It Me?

When conflict arises, the first question I ask myself is: am I the problem?

This isn't about self-blame. It's about objective assessment. Did I contribute to this conflict? Is there something I did or didn't do that created this situation? Is there something about my approach or my communication that's causing the issue?

So far, in my advocacy work, I don't think I've been the problem. But that's only because I'm constantly asking myself that question. I'm constantly examining the situation objectively.

This requires honest self-reflection. It requires willingness to admit fault. It requires not being defensive when someone gives you feedback.

If you're always right, you'll never learn. You'll never grow. You'll never understand what's actually happening in conflict situations.

But if you're willing to ask yourself: "Is this me?", you create space for real learning. You create space for resolution.

What Makes Conflicts Resolvable

When I think about conflicts I've heard about or observed from a distance, I notice the ones that get resolved have something in common: they don't turn into permanent rifts.

The people involved are honest and straightforward. They're not playing games. They're not being passive-aggressive. They're not trying to manipulate or control the situation.

They're also not bringing emotion and bias into the conversation. They're not letting personal feelings drive the discussion. They're staying focused on the issue.

And critically, the other party is willing to listen. They're willing to hear feedback. They're willing to consider a different perspective. They're willing to change if change is warranted.

When both sides show up with honesty, straightforwardness, and willingness to listen, conflicts can be resolved. Relationships can be repaired. Understanding can be reached.

When one or both sides are defensive, emotional, or unwilling to listen, conflicts fester. They grow. They become permanent.

This is why the foundation of conflict resolution is the same as the foundation of good advocacy: authenticity, clarity, and respect.

Avoiding Conflict Through Clear Communication

The best way to handle conflict is to avoid unnecessary conflict in the first place.

This means communicating clearly about expectations. It means asking questions instead of making assumptions. It means checking in when something feels off.

It means being direct about feedback instead of letting resentment build. It means having difficult conversations early, before they become crises.

It means approaching people with good faith. Assuming they want to do well. Assuming their intentions are good unless proven otherwise.

Most of the time, conflict comes from misunderstanding. Someone said something that landed wrong. Someone didn't understand what was being asked. Someone's expectations weren't aligned with reality.

Clear communication prevents a lot of that. It doesn't prevent all conflict. But it prevents the kind of unnecessary conflict that poisons relationships.

When to Walk Away

Sometimes, despite your best efforts to communicate clearly and resolve conflict, the situation doesn't improve.

Sometimes an organization isn't interested in feedback. Sometimes an advocate isn't interested in change. Sometimes the relationship just isn't healthy.

In those cases, the answer is to walk away.

This doesn't mean making a dramatic exit or burning bridges publicly. It means making a quiet decision to stop collaborating. To stop showing up. To redirect your energy toward relationships and work that are healthier.

You don't owe anyone your participation. You don't owe an organization your advocacy. You don't owe a relationship if it's not serving you or the mission.

Walking away can be an act of integrity. It can be honoring your own boundaries. It can be making space for someone else who might be a better fit.

The Bottom Line

Conflict in advocacy work is inevitable. But how you handle it deter-mines whether it becomes a growth opportunity or a permanent rupture.

Approach conflicts with honesty. Approach them with clarity. Approach them with the assumption that the other person has good intentions. Ask yourself if you're the problem. Be willing to listen. Be willing to change if change is warranted.

And when resolution isn't possible, have the integrity to walk away.

Most of the time, that approach will serve you well. It will help you navigate the complex relationships that advocacy work requires. It will help you maintain the integrity that makes advocacy powerful in the first place.

Because at the end of the day, advocacy is about serving patients and creating change. When conflict gets in the way of that mission, it's time to address it. And when it can't be addressed, it's time to move on.

Chapter 17
The Future of Healthcare Advocacy

Healthcare advocacy is at an inflection point. The field has matured dramatically over the past decade. Patient voices are more valued. Research is becoming more patient-centered. Organizations are starting to recognize that authentic advocacy strengthens their work.

But we're only at the beginning. The future of healthcare advocacy will be shaped by how we respond to the opportunities and challenges ahead.

Patients at the Center

Healthcare advocacy is evolving from a model where patients are centered in research and decision-making to one where they are true partners. I believe we are heading toward a future where patients are not merely consulted, nor simply centered, but genuinely partnered in the work of research.

With the growth of AI and advanced technology in research, the patient perspective will be even more important. Why? Because patients bring something technology can't replicate: lived experience.

The human reality of navigating disease. The barriers that data alone can't capture. The priorities that matter in real life, not just in clinical trials.

As research becomes more sophisticated, the need for grounding that research in patient reality becomes more critical. AI can process massive amounts of data. But it takes a patient to say: "This treatment works, but the side effects make it impossible to work. That matters more than what you're measuring."

Patient-centered research hasn't really become a thing until the past decade. And we still have a long way to go. But the trajectory is clear. Patients will be more central to research design, implementation, and interpretation.

The Critical Role of Advocacy in a Tech-Driven World

Because of the advancements in technology, it will be even more important for advocates to ensure their voices are heard. Not less. More.

Here's why: technology is designed by humans. And humans are biased. By nature, we are biased. We bring our perspectives, our experiences, our blind spots into the tools we create.

When AI is used in research or healthcare, it's reflecting the biases of the people who built it and the data it was trained on. When digital platforms are used for patient engagement, they're designed with certain assumptions about how people interact and communicate.

Patient advocates are essential to identifying and correcting those biases. To pushing back on technology that doesn't serve patients. To demanding that innovation happens with patient input, not just for patients.

This is why diversity and inclusion in advocacy spaces is so critical. Different perspectives catch different biases. Different cultural norms, religious beliefs, and lived experiences reveal blind spots that homogeneous groups never would.

We need more diversity in advocacy. More voices from communities historically excluded from healthcare research and decision-making. More representation that reflects the full complexity of patient experience.

And we need this even—maybe especially—in a period where DEI programs are being slashed and penalized. When the broader culture is moving away from diversity work, advocacy spaces need to double down on it. Because the stakes for patients are too high to do otherwise.

Playing the Long Game

With the way politics has become, playing the long game is more important than ever. Which takes commitment and consistency.

We saw this with the Medicare Part D reforms. It took a decade of sustained advocacy. Year after year of showing up. Of telling stories. Of building relationships. Of not giving up even when nothing seemed to be changing.

That long game is harder in today's political environment. Everything moves faster. Attention spans are shorter. There's pressure for immediate results.

But the most meaningful change still takes time. It takes organizations and advocates who are willing to stay committed. It takes playing the long game even when the short-term wins feel distant.

This is one of the reasons why organizational commitment to advocacy matters so much. Because individual advocates can't sustain the long game alone. They need organizations backing them. They need funding. They need structure. They need community.

Challenges as Opportunities

I'm a big believer that we can look at anything as a problem or opportunity. And I choose to see the challenges ahead as opportunities in disguise.

The challenge of increasing politicization in healthcare? An opportunity to build advocacy that's so rooted in patient benefit that it transcends politics.

The challenge of AI and technology in healthcare? An opportunity to ensure patient voices shape how technology is developed and implemented.

The challenge of limited resources? An opportunity to be more strategic about how advocacy funding is allocated.

The challenge of diverse perspectives sometimes conflicting? An opportunity to build stronger consensus because we've actually heard and integrated different viewpoints.

Every obstacle is an invitation to think differently. To approach the work from a new angle. To build something better than what existed before.

The Evolving Role of Patient Advocates

The role of the patient advocate is evolving. And it's shifting in a fundamental way.

For a long time, being asked to participate in advocacy felt like an honor. You were honored to be at the table. You were grateful for the opportunity. You questioned whether you belonged there.

That's changing. The future is where patient advocates question when they aren't at the table. Where it becomes expected that patients are involved in research design. Where organizations that don't have patient input are the outliers, not the norm.

This shift reflects growing recognition that patient advocacy isn't a nice-to-have. It's essential. It's fundamental to how healthcare research and policy should work.

As more advocates internalize this, as more organizations recognize this, the role of the advocate becomes stronger. More central. More valued.

Barriers Need to Come Down

If we're serious about advancing healthcare advocacy, we need to lower the barriers to getting involved.

Right now, advocacy is often accessible to people with certain privileges. People with flexible work schedules. People without caregiving responsibilities. People with financial stability. People with transportation. People who speak English fluently.

We need to ask: who is excluded by our current approach to advocacy? And then we need to change the approach.

This might mean providing compensation so people don't have to volunteer. It might mean offering virtual participation options. It might mean providing childcare at events. It might mean translating materials into multiple languages. It might mean meeting people where they are, rather than asking them to come to us.

Lowering barriers takes resources. It takes commitment. But it's essential if we want advocacy that truly represents all patients, not just the ones with privilege.

More Resources, Better Funding

Patient-centered research and advocacy require resources. More resources than are currently being invested.

Researchers need to budget for compensating patient partners. Organizations need dedicated staff for patient engagement. Advocates need support to sustain their work over time.

Right now, much advocacy work happens because people are passionate and volunteer their time. That's beautiful. But it's not sustainable. And it's not equitable. It expects unpaid labor from people who are already managing illness or recovery.

The future of advocacy requires more funding explicitly tied to patient-centered work. Funding for training and education. Funding for compensation. Funding for infrastructure that supports advocates.

This isn't just good for advocates. It's good for the research and policy work itself. Because when advocates are supported, when they're compensated fairly, when they have resources behind them, they can do better work. Deeper work. More strategic work.

The Vision: An Advocate Union

This is where my vision for the future comes in. I envision an Advocate Union.

A place where all healthcare advocates can receive training and education. Where they learn not just about their specific disease or condition, but about how healthcare advocacy works. How research works. How policy works. How to be effective in different advocacy contexts.

A place where advocates are connected with research projects and legislative efforts. Where they don't have to search for opportunities or wait to be discovered. Where opportunities come to them because the union matches advocates with needs.

A place where advocates sit on steering committees, boards, and advisory panels. Where they have a collective voice that organizations can't ignore.

A place where advocates are compensated fairly for their time and expertise. Where they're not taken advantage of. Where the value of their work is recognized financially.

An Advocate Union wouldn't compete with existing organizations like Fight CRC or PAN Foundation. It would complement them. It would create infrastructure that supports all advocacy work. It would ensure that no advocate falls through the cracks. It would democratize access to advocacy training and opportunities.

Right now, if you're lucky, you might find an organization that mentors you. If you're not, you figure it out on your own. An Advocate Union would remove that luck factor.

It would also give advocates collective power. A union is stronger than individuals. It can advocate for better treatment of patient advisors. It can set standards for compensation. It can push back against organizations that try to exploit patient voices.

What Needs to Change

For this future to become reality, some things need to shift.

Healthcare organizations need to stop seeing patient advocacy as optional. It needs to be fundamental to how they operate. Built into budgets. Built into timelines. Built into decision-making from the start.

Research institutions need to invest in patient-centered approaches. Not as an add-on. As core methodology.

Funders need to prioritize patient-centered research and advocacy infrastructure. Not just disease research or treatment development. But the structures and support systems that make patient engagement possible.

Policymakers need to recognize that patient voices strengthen policy. That patient input leads to better outcomes. That advocacy isn't special interest lobbying. It's the voice of people who are most affected by policy decisions.

And advocates need to expect more for themselves. To demand fair compensation. To expect organizations to listen. To question when they're not at the table. To build collective power.

A Decade of Progress, Infinite Room for Growth

We've made enormous progress in the past decade. Patient-centered research has emerged from a fringe idea to becoming mainstream. Advocacy organizations have professionalized. More organizations are taking patient input seriously.

But we're still in the early stages. We're still proving something that should be obvious: that patients have expertise worth paying for.

The future of healthcare advocacy is bright. But it requires sustained effort. It requires commitment. It requires people willing to keep pushing even when the system resists.

It requires you. Whether you're a newly diagnosed patient wondering if your voice matters, a seasoned advocate ready to push for systemic change, or an organization realizing that authentic patient engagement will strengthen your work.

The future of healthcare advocacy is being built right now. By advocates who show up. By organizations that listen. By researchers who center patient voices. By funders who prioritize patient-centered work.

It's being built by you. Keep building it. Keep pushing. Keep advocating.

Because the future where patients are truly centered in healthcare? That future is within reach. But only if we all commit to making it real.

Conclusion: Your Advocacy Mandate

When I heard those three words — "you have cancer" — advocacy wasn't part of my plan. I was focused on survival, on treatment options, on simply getting through each day. But along this journey, I discovered something powerful: my story matters. And sharing it became the foundation of my advocacy.

That discovery changed everything. It transformed me from a patient navigating a disease into an advocate working to change systems. It gave me purpose. It gave me power.

And it can for you too.

The Core Truth

Throughout this book, we've talked about different types of advocacy. About how to build your voice. About how to work with organizations. About how to sustain yourself in this work.

But underneath all of that is a single, simple truth:

Your story matters. And when you share it, you create change.

Change doesn't always come in the form you expect. It doesn't always happen on your timeline. But when patients decide to speak up, when they refuse to stay silent about their experiences, when they insist on being partners in healthcare decisions—that's when systems shift.

We've seen it happen. Screening age recommendations changing. Medicare reforms passing after a decade of advocacy. Research studies becoming more patient-centered. Organizations recognizing that genuine patient engagement strengthens their work.

All of that started with individual patients deciding their voices mattered. Deciding to share their stories. Deciding to advocate.

Moving From Patient-Centered to Patient as Partner

Throughout this book, I've talked about the shift from patient-centered care and research to patients being true partners. That's the future we're building.

Patient-centered means your needs are considered. It's an improvement over ignoring patients entirely.

But patient as partner means something different. It means you're at the table from the beginning. It means your voice shapes decisions. It means you're not just informed about what's happening—you're actively creating what happens next.

This isn't a subtle difference. It's fundamental. It changes the power dynamic. It changes who decides what matters. It changes outcomes.

And this shift only happens when patients demand it. When advocates insist on partnership instead of consultation. When organizations recognize that patients bring irreplaceable expertise.

You can be part of that shift. In fact, you are part of that shift, whether you recognize it or not.

For the Newly Diagnosed

If you're reading this book because you've just been diagnosed, let me say something first: I'm sorry. I know how overwhelming this is. I know how much fear lives in your body right now.

You don't have to be an advocate. You don't have to do anything beyond taking care of yourself and getting the treatment you need.

But I want you to know something: don't let the word "advocacy" scare you. It sounds big and important, and like something other people do.

Advocacy is just sharing your story. It's telling someone newly diagnosed what you wish you'd known. It's asking your doctor the hard questions. It's connecting with others who understand. It's deciding that your experience matters and that you're going to say so.

That's advocacy. And you can start today.

Start where you are. You don't need credentials. You don't need permission. You just need to be willing to share your experience.

Tell your story on social media if that feels right. Connect with a support group. Reach out to an advocacy organization. Contact your elected representatives. Participate in research if an opportunity comes up.

You'll be amazed at what happens when you decide your voice matters.

For Current Advocates

If you're already engaged with this work, I have different questions for you:

What are you passionate about? What type of advocacy makes you feel alive rather than drained? Where do you want to go next?

Too many advocates spread themselves thin. They say yes to every-thing. They burn out. They lose the work that fueled them.

Instead, I'm asking you to get strategic. To understand what energizes you. To focus your efforts there. To make a bigger impact in the areas where you're most committed.

And then, I'm asking you to inspire others. To mentor newly diagnosed patients. To show them that their voice matters. To build the next generation of advocates.

Because this movement only grows when advocates like you pull others in. When you model what it looks like to sustain this work. When you show that advocacy isn't something you have to sacrifice everything for—it's something you can do alongside your life.

Be the advocate you needed when you were newly diagnosed. Mentor others. Build community. And then push your own work further.

For Organizations

If you're leading an organization serving patients, I have a question for you:

How are you treating your advocates right now? Are you using them or empowering them?

There's a difference. Using advocates means extracting their stories, their time, their expertise. It means asking for their input but not actually listening. It means checking a box so you can say you have patient engagement.

Empowering advocates means something different. It means compensating them fairly. It means listening to their feedback and acting on it. It means giving them real authority in decision-making. It means supporting them through the emotional toll of this work. It means recognizing them publicly for their contributions.

The organizations that succeed are the ones that invest in authentic patient engagement. Not as an add-on. As core to how they operate.

If you're not doing that yet, start now. Ask your patient advisors what they need. Compensate them. Listen to their feedback. Change based on what you hear. Report the impact back to them so they see their work mattering.

Your organization will be stronger for it. Your advocates will be more engaged. Your impact will deepen.

For Policymakers and Funders

When you're making decisions about healthcare policy or funding research, remember this: patients are not just beneficiaries of your decisions. They are experts. They bring knowledge that no researcher, no clinician, no policymaker can match.

Make sure patients are part of the process. Not as an afterthought. Not as a consultation after decisions are already made. But as partners from the beginning.

When you fund research, require that it includes authentic patient engagement. When you make policy, make sure patients shaped that policy. When you allocate resources, ensure that patient-centered work is prioritized.

The patients affected by your decisions should be the ones helping make those decisions. Not because it's nice. But because it makes the work better.

The Vision: An Advocate Union

Now, I want to paint a picture of what the future could look like.

Imagine an Advocate Union. A place where healthcare advocates can get training and education. Where they learn not just about their disease, but about how advocacy works. How research works. How policy works.

A place where advocates are connected with research projects and legislative efforts. Where opportunities come to them. Where they can find the advocacy work that matches their passion and capacity.

A place where advocates sit on steering committees, boards, and advisory panels. Where they have collective voice that organizations can't ignore.

A place where advocates are compensated fairly for their time and expertise. Where they're not taken advantage of. Where the value of their work is recognized financially.

A place where newly diagnosed patients can turn and ask: "How do I get involved?" And have clear, accessible pathways to answer that question.

This Advocate Union wouldn't replace organizations like Fight CRC or PAN Foundation. It would complement them. It would create infrastructure that supports all advocacy work. It would ensure that no advocate falls through the cracks. It would democratize access to advocacy.

And it would give advocates collective power. Power to push back against exploitation. Power to set standards for how they're treated. Power to demand that organizations take patient engagement seriously.

This vision is possible. But only if we build it together.

Your Advocacy Mandate

I'm not asking you to become an advocate if you don't want to. I'm not asking you to burn yourself out. I'm not asking you to sacrifice your health or wellbeing.

But I am asking you to recognize the power you hold. Your story has the capacity to change someone's life. Your voice has the capacity to influence policy. Your participation in research can shape the future of treatment.

That's not an exaggeration. That's not me being inspirational for the sake of it. That's reality.

So, here's my mandate for you:

If you're newly diagnosed: Don't let the word "advocacy" scare you. Understand the power of sharing your story. Start where you are. Tell your truth. Connect with others. Your voice matters.

If you're already an advocate: What are you passionate about? How can you move further in that direction and make a bigger impact? How can you inspire others to become advocates? Don't burn out trying to do everything. Focus on what fuels you and deepen that work.

If you're leading an organization: How are you treating your advocates now? Are you using them or empowering them? How can you empower them even more? What barriers exist to their full participation, and how will you remove them?

If you're a policymaker or funder: Make sure patients are part of the process. Not just a number. Not just a beneficiary. A partner. An expert. Someone whose voice shapes what happens next.

The Work Continues

This book is a guide for the journey ahead. But it's not the end of the story. The work of advocacy continues. The building of systems that truly center patients as partners continues. The creation of an Advocate Union continues.

And it continues because of people like you. People who read this book and realized their voice matters. People who decided to share their stories. People who insisted on being partners in healthcare. People who refused to accept systems that ignore patient expertise.

I don't know what your specific role in this movement will be. Maybe you'll become a fierce legislative advocate. Maybe you'll mentor newly diagnosed patients. Maybe you'll serve on research committees. Maybe you'll do something I haven't even imagined yet.

But I know this: your voice matters. Your experience matters. And in sharing your story, you're already creating change.

The future where patients are true partners in healthcare? That future is within reach. It's being built right now by advocates willing to show up.

Keep building it. Keep pushing. Keep advocating.

Because the world needs your voice. And patients need to know they're not alone.

Your advocacy mandate is simple: share your story. Build community. Demand partnership. Inspire others.

That's how we create the future we all deserve. Welcome to the movement.

Notes

What is Advocacy? Defining Your Why

1. Copp, L.A. (1986). "The nurse as advocate for vulnerable persons." Journal of Advanced Nursing, 11, 255-263. As cited in: Journal of Cancer Policy, Volume 35 (2023), which defines patient advocacy as "the act of representing and pleading on behalf of patients to ensure their rights are upheld and improve access to quality treatment and care." https://www.sciencedirect.com/science/article/abs/pii/ S2213538323000309

The Evolution of Healthcare Advocacy as an Industry

1. Hibbard JH, Greene J. "What the evidence shows about patient activation: better health outcomes and care experiences; fewer data on costs." Health Aff (Millwood). 2013 Feb;32(2):207-14.

2. Centers for Disease Control and Prevention. "Patient Engagement: Health Outcomes and Cost." Health Literacy Research Summaries. https://www.cdc.gov/ health-literacy/php/research-summaries/patient-engagement.html. Accessed January 2026. Citing: Greene J, Hibbard JH, Sacks R, Overton V, Parrotta CD. "When patient activation levels change, health outcomes and costs change, too." Health Aff (Millwood). 2015 Mar;34(3):431-7. doi: 10.1377/hlthaff.2014.0452.

About the Author

Tim McDonald is a healthcare advocate with five years of experience focused on colorectal cancer. His roles include serving as a Research Advocate with Fight CRC, Florida Chapter Leader for Man Up To Cancer, and member of HOPA's Patient Advisory Council. He also serves on the Patient and Family Advisory Council for the PAN Foun-dation, is a PCORI Ambassador, and holds a leadership position within the COLONTOWN community. Beyond these roles, Tim hosts the Advocacy at Work podcast and brings 17 years of community management experience to his advocacy practice. He has presented on advocacy and community building across the United States, Canada, Mexico, and Europe.

Learn more about Tim's work at AdvocacyAtWork.com and connect with him on LinkedIn.